FINDING AND REVEALING YOUR SEXUAL SELF

FINDING AND REVEALING YOUR SEXUAL SELF

A Guide to Communicating about Sex

Libby Bennett and Ginger Holczer

ROWMAN & LITTLEFIELD PUBLISHERS, INC.
Lanham • Boulder • New York • Toronto • Plymouth, UK

Published by Rowman & Littlefield Publishers, Inc.
A wholly owned subsidiary of The Rowman & Littlefield Publishing Group, Inc.
4501 Forbes Boulevard, Suite 200, Lanham, Maryland 20706
http://www.rowmanlittlefield.com

Estover Road, Plymouth PL6 7PY, United Kingdom

British Library Cataloguing in Publication Information Available

Library of Congress Cataloging-in-Publication Data
Bennett, Libby, 1958-
  Finding and revealing your sexual self : a guide to communicating about sex
/ Libby Bennett and Ginger Holczer.
     p. cm.
  Includes bibliographical references.
  ISBN 978-1-4422-0036-4 (cloth : alk. paper)
  1. Communication in sex. I. Holczer, Ginger, 1960- II. Title.
  HQ23.B44 2010
  306.7—dc22   2009042612

∞™ The paper used in this publication meets the minimum requirements of
American National Standard for Information Sciences—Permanence of Paper
for Printed Library Materials, ANSI/NISO Z39.48-1992.

Printed in the United States of America

This book is dedicated to all of our clients who had the courage to share the struggles of their relationships and taught us the intricacy of human sexuality.

CONTENTS

ACKNOWLEDGMENTS

We are grateful to many people who have helped with the creation of our book. We will only be able to mention some by name, but we're thankful to so many who encouraged and supported us over the years with the concept of this book.

Foremost, our thanks go to Suzanne Staszak-Silva and the staff at Rowman & Littlefield for believing in us, new authors to this great publishing company. Suzanne, your friendly, lightning-quick responses gave us guidance and hope when we found ourselves questioning our writing or direction.

Our colleagues at the office have also been there to encourage us. Special heartfelt thanks go to Dr. Kathy LeMon, who has been a mentor to us both and enthusiastically supported us in every one of our endeavors. We don't want to forget Hal Davidson, who moved on from our office but is still in our hearts. We learned so much about human sexuality and keeping a sense of humor from Hal.

To our office staff, DeAnna and Emily, we are forever grateful! You are two beautiful women, both inside and out. You keep us running with precision, support, and great humor.

We are indebted to the sex therapists, counselors, and educators of AASECT, an amazing group of people. They have provided us with invaluable books, DVDs, conferences, listserv insights, workshops, and conversations that allowed us to pursue our dream of writing this book.

From Libby: I want to thank Dr. Ginger Holczer, my coauthor, office-mate, and friend. We have taken on so many endeavors, and this one has been an amazing journey! We shared the driving, navigated together through the muck, and always made the final stop in wine country. I'm glad to have made the trip with you!

Special thanks go to Dr. Mark Skrade, the president of Forest Institute, who encouraged me to pursue my certification in sex therapy. The certification has introduced me to many valuable therapeutic tools and wonderful friends through AASECT, and it has allowed me to teach and present in the exciting field of human sexuality.

On a personal note, I want to thank my parents, sister, and friends, who have believed in me and loved me over the years. I am grateful for your encouragement and support. Asante sana! Jon Davis, thank you for cheering me on. My deepest appreciation will always be for my two children, Ryan and Ellen. You have been my greatest inspiration for creation, passion, and strength. Your love, wit, intelligence, and sweet hugs are my dearest treasure.

From Ginger: I would like to thank my partner in this endeavor, Dr. Libby Bennett, who worked so diligently to make sure all the details were attended to for the book. Thanks for the skeleton that made this book a reality for us, and for letting me be part of such a wonderful experience. Thanks for feeding me every weekend, and for the evening "wine tastings." I'm glad we were able to become such good friends and can't wait to see what the future holds for us!

Thanks to my mentors, Dr. AnnElise Parkhurst and the late Dr. Robert Murney, who taught me in so many words that not only was sex okay to discuss in therapy, but *must* be discussed in therapy.

Big thanks to my parents and brother for always encouraging my academic pursuits, and to my extended family for being my cheerleaders. Thanks to my friends who allowed themselves to be put on the back burner while we worked on the book. Special thanks to Aunt Peg for listening and understanding throughout the years.

To Corey, Katy, Brent, Emily, Justin, Lacey, Tyler, Wyatt, and Llewellyn; you are the center of my world—thanks for your undying love and support. You provide me with so many laughs and such love for life! Lastly, to my partner Tom, who picked up the slack in our lives during the time Libby and I were busy writing. Thanks for going on this journey with me even when the path was unsure and scary. I can't think of anyone I'd rather have walking beside me.

1

ARE YOU TALKING TO YOURSELF?

Sometimes I feel like I don't know myself very well. When I was growing up, my family didn't talk about sex, and I'm not sure I know what I want for myself sexually.

—Female, age 36

①

SPEAKING OF SEX

Beginning the Journey

We have avoided talking about sex for so long now; I don't know where to start.

—Male, age 40

- Are you able to talk easily about sex?
- Do you hope your sexual problems will "just go away"?
- Can you acknowledge your differences as a couple?
- Do you avoid each other sexually and physically?
- Are you able talk to your doctor or therapist about sex?

We see it on the "big screen": two lovers, falling in the sand, waves crashing over them, bodies entwined . . . it all looks so erotic and effortless! In real bedrooms, everyone else has to wrestle with experiences that aren't quite so sexy: flaccid penises, low desire, ejaculating too soon, vaginal pain, and more! These problems can't be ignored, but how do we talk about them? Erotic life is complex, and talking about it can be awkward and scary. Without the skills to communicate about sex, a relationship will likely become disconnected, frustrating, and even downright boring! So join us for an intimate conversation about a very personal topic . . . sex!

Suzanne and Sam,* a couple in their early fifties, came to therapy to talk about their sexual desire discrepancy. Sam noticed his sex drive was low, which was a change for him. Suzanne also discovered some changes about herself and talked with her gynecologist about her waning sex drive and the changes of menopause. The doctor suggested a vaginal moisturizer and estrogen cream. Suzanne's libido began to return and she found herself with increased sexual desire. Sam admitted that he had erectile changes and these changes were very discouraging. He feared attempting intercourse, having realized that he could not count on his erection being as firm as it had been when he was young. Their therapist educated Sam and Suzanne about the normal physical changes for males and females as they age. As they discussed and learned about their changing bodies and needs, Suzanne and Sam both began to relax regarding the expectation of performance. They found that being able to communicate honestly about the challenges of aging brought relief and a revitalized sexual relationship.

WHY WRITE *ANOTHER* BOOK ABOUT SEX?

As sex and relationship therapists, we are constantly engaged with individuals and couples struggling to find their sexual voices. Every day, we hear distress and confusion as people try to sort through their thoughts and feelings about sex. In order to help our clients find resources, we began looking for material about sexual communication. We found that most of the books begin in the bedroom, even under the sheets! There are books about increasing desire, having better sex, unusual sexual positions, and other topics that are either too steamy or too clinical for our clients. We read these books and recommended them, but none really fit the bill.

We began holding small group sessions and seminars for women about their sexual selves. We held workshops for therapists and healthcare providers about the sexual needs of their clients. We spoke to community groups about sexuality and aging, sexuality and cancer, and plain

---

*Suzanne and Sam, as well as all of the other examples mentioned in this book, come from our therapy practices, but we have changed the names and identifying details to protect confidentiality.

ol' sexuality. Along the way, many people told us that they appreciated our "no-holds-barred" discussions about sex and enjoyed the humor we used.

Our clients told us that they were having difficulty bringing up their sexual concerns to those in the helping profession and that therapists weren't asking.

Michael and Marcie came to the office for therapy, after fifteen years in their relationship and three other therapy experiences. During the second session, the therapist asked the couple about their sexual encounters. After a pause, Michael admitted that sex was a big part of what was bothering him about the relationship. Michael went on to say that he missed the intimate connection he had had with Marcie and felt as though she was no longer attracted to him. The therapist was able to discuss the issue in therapy, and worked with them on the sexual part of their intimacy. Marcie assured Michael that she was physically attracted to him, and that "life just seems to get in the way, sometimes." Michael grew tearful at the end of the therapy session, telling the therapist that in all the years they had sought marital therapy, not once were they asked about sex.

This is a story that we have heard over and over again in our practice. People have difficulty discussing sex with their partners, with their therapists, and also with their medical doctors.

Katrina and Kathy came to therapy talking about Kathy's interest in other women. They disclosed that they have been together for ten years, and during the ten years Katrina has been on an antidepressant that lowered her sexual desire. She found herself turning down sex with Kathy on a regular basis. Her doctor never told her about this particular side effect of the medication, and Katrina came across this information on the Internet. But the damage had been done. The couple had gotten into a pattern of Katrina avoiding sex and Kathy seeking sex elsewhere. Of course, this is no excuse for Kathy, but a conversation with Katrina, Kathy, and the doctor might have given Katrina other options. Other medications or treatments might not have had this kind of side effect.

In workshops for health-care providers, we heard them struggling with how to talk about the touchy subject of their patients' sexual concerns.

Dr. Johnson spoke to us after our presentation regarding female sexual disorders, "I really need some tools to discuss these issues with my female patients. Listening to you, I felt like you were sitting in my office hearing my patients talk about their concerns. Thank you for bringing this to our conference because we need to connect with our patients about this topic!"

So, we put our heads together and decided to write about sex. We want to address the topic of sex, which still leaves so many of us with our tongues tied and our faces blushing.

WHY READ *ANOTHER* BOOK ABOUT SEX?

We want you to be able to understand your own sexuality, learn about your partner's, and then express it to your partner and professionals, if necessary. The book is divided into three parts that will aid you in the journey to know your sexual self and then express that self to others. The first section, "Are You Talking to Yourself?" leads you to explore your past and your own uniqueness. The second section, "Are You Talking to Me?" gives strategies to communicate sexual needs, negotiate the rough waters in a relationship, and fan the flames of sexuality. Finally, "Is Anyone Listening?" provides helpful information for communicating with a therapist or physician. The "Sexual Healing" sections of the book provide questions and answers regarding sexual concerns. Although the identifying information has been changed in the "Sexual Healing" questions to protect the confidentiality of our clients, these are concerns we have heard from people in our private practices and speaking engagements.

The Bridge to Sexual Awareness

The journey to better communication about sex is one that we visualize taking place on a bridge. The journey begins with the desire to know the depth of one's own sexuality. There are many factors that make up the path across the bridge. Some relate to individual sexuality: childhood perceptions, sexual wounds, sexual uniqueness, and life-stage challenges. Others relate to one's relationship with a partner, such as communication, expectations, relationship struggles, and desire. These individual and relationship components lead to sexual awareness. Being able to talk about these issues will help a person get his or her sexual voice heard.

BUT WHY DO I NEED TO *TALK* ABOUT SEX?

It seems that there's a lot of talk about talk! *Oprah* and *Dr. Phil* do it. There are books everywhere about it. So, why all this emphasis on talking?

As therapists, we understand that some people aren't comfortable having conversations. Especially about sex! We hear the discomfort in our private practice, at seminars, and in our own personal relationships. We know that, without someone bringing up the subject of sex, a lot of important issues start simmering on the back burner until things come to a boiling point.

 SEXUAL HEALING

Why is it important to understand myself in order to communicate about sex? I don't feel that my sexual problems are just *my* problem, I feel like it's *our* problem. And my partner has issues too!

It's necessary to know yourself before you can communicate that knowledge to someone else. When talking about sex, understanding where your ideas and perceptions came from can be helpful as you express yourself to someone else. You can't have a conversation without both knowing where you came from and where you want to go. We agree that sexual issues for a couple is an "our" problem. But you need to begin with self-understanding.

AND *HOW* DO I TALK ABOUT SEX?

Communication is an essential part of a relationship. When thoughts and feelings are expressed accurately and heard with empathy, it's possible to grow closer, feel safer, and develop deeper intimacy. Responding in a respectful manner will create an environment where there is a freedom for expression. Start intimate conversations slowly, remembering to keep a sense of humor, and be aware of positive and negative reactions.

Keep in mind that a safe place is needed to have conversations about sex, and a relationship is not always a safe harbor. There may be some wounds from the past that need to be fixed in order to get to a place where there is a sense of security. If the relationship feels physically or emotionally unsafe, professional help may be necessary to increase understanding in order to feel more secure and form a more satisfying sexual bond. There's more about safety in chapter 6.

We want to encourage open communication regarding sexual needs, fears, and desires. Be assured that we will move slowly and provide many examples throughout this book. When there are sexual communication problems, it's safe to say that other areas of communication are suffering, too. Communication promotes connectedness, but when you aren't connected, it can seem like your partner is speaking a foreign language.

> Tyler and Tessa, a young couple in their twenties, came to see the therapist with little to say initially. Tessa asked Tyler to explain why they were in therapy and she sat and listened to her partner, with her arms crossed over her chest. Tyler looked very uncomfortable as he explained that he had been dealing with rapid ejaculation for the entire two years of their relationship. They weren't able to talk about this at home without ending up in tears and fighting. Tyler blamed himself, and Tessa felt frustrated and hopeless. Tessa and Tyler's sexual issues had permeated their relationship in other ways, as well. The tension of the unresolved sexual problem followed them into their interactions with each other as they attempted to discuss money and time management. Because they did not feel like intimate partners in the bedroom, they also didn't feel close and connected in other areas of their relationship. Both Tessa and Tyler disliked the confrontations and began to avoid talking, touching, or planning time with each other. After several months of learning effective communication, they were able to talk to each other about their sexual concerns, which led them to feel more connected and compatible.

We'll go more fully into the art of communication in chapter 6, but here are some points to consider as you read this book:

Tips for Communicating with Your Partner

- Listening is something that takes practice. Most of us have trouble hearing the other person because we are preparing our own rebuttal.
- You and your partner are different. Don't expect agreement. Expect diversity.
- Simply venting your anger may make you feel better or bigger, but it won't help your relationship. Try to express yourself, but also be kind and not threatening.
- Keep your statements to a minimum. Your partner can't hold on to too much information. It becomes overwhelming.
- Ask specific questions if you need clarification.
- Stay away from generalizations such as, "You always . . ." or "You never . . ."
- Time-out is a good tool, as long as you and your partner agree to the rules and come back to the issue later.
- Agree on how to keep your conversation private. Is it okay to talk to your best friend or your brother about your sexual issues?
- Try paraphrasing what the other said. Check to see if you heard your partner correctly.
- Express empathy for what your partner is feeling. Empathy doesn't mean that you agree with their statement or opinion. Empathy shows compassion, validation, and understanding.
- Use "I feel" statements. Don't assume that you know what your partner feels. Avoid "you" statements.
- Mind reading works only at the state fair! Check things out with each other. Remember that you're not the expert on your partner.

SEX . . . LOVE . . .
WHAT'S MY BRAIN HAVE TO DO WITH IT?

This book is intended to help people connect and communicate about sex despite differences such as childhood, uniqueness, and personal challenges. But what about our chemical makeup? Other than some gender differences, chemically we appear to be quite similar.

Why do we fall in love and desire sexual intimacy? It's helpful to explore the ebb and flow of love in order to communicate about changes in our sexual relationships. Understanding the neuroscience behind "falling in love" can help us make sense of the powerful emotional and sexual drives experienced in long-term relationships.

There appear to be three separate systems that play a part in this thing called love. The first system or drive, *lust*, is fueled primarily by testosterone for both men and women. We are driven by hormones and chemicals deep within primitive brain structures to seek sexual partners.

The second system, *romantic love*, is discussed in Helen Fisher's book, *Why We Love*, in which she reports on studies that use neuroimaging to pinpoint the chemicals in the brain associated with this system.[1] The stage of romantic love, in which the couple focuses its energy exclusively and intensely on one another, usually lasts about six to eighteen months. Scanning with functional magnetic resonance imaging (fMRI) has indicated that individuals who were looking at a photo of their "beloved" had significantly elevated activity in the brain area known as the ventral tegmental area. Cells in this area of the brain distribute dopamine, a neurotransmitter that drives us to seek what is necessary for survival, for example, food, water, and sex. Dopamine is distributed to different parts of the brain, allowing us to focus and concentrate on pursuing a reward, as well as producing a great deal of energy and "feelings of elation." When the object of desire is found, there is a sense of intense reward, even a high, which motivates us to continue our pursuit for more. Dopamine often drives up the hormone testosterone, resulting in the desire for sex.

The third system is called *attachment* or *companionate love* and cements the bond of the relationship. Neuroscience has shown that this stage occurs gradually and appears to be facilitated primarily by two hormones, oxytocin and vasopressin, that flood the brain during intimate connections. This reaction tends to affect dopamine and norepinephrine activity in the brain, reducing the effects of romantic love and causing the wave of excitation that occurs when we first "hook up" to wane.

As noted above, the romantic stage in any relationship naturally fades. How many times have affairs been fueled by this intense heady feeling of "love," only to find that it disappears with time. It's understandable that we become distressed when we feel the sexual thrill is gone. Chapter 9 contains more information about techniques to stimulate and invigorate a sexual relationship that has lost its fire.

HOW TO USE THIS BOOK

This book is first and foremost about communication and is written for couples—straight, gay, lesbian, bisexual, or transgender. The information can be used by partners, whether married, dating, or living together. Although we have written the book to be sensitive to and inclusive of *all* relationships, straight or otherwise, there are resources at the end of this book that will address specific issues more fully. If you are not in a relationship, this book can be helpful as you prepare for a relationship or do a "mental autopsy" on a past relationship.

Our book gives "sexercises," to engage you in exploring your sexuality, enhancing your communication, and increasing your intimacy and passion. Throughout the book, we have included examples of individuals, just like you, who are struggling with understanding and expressing their sexual concerns. The "Sexual Healing" sections of the book answer specific questions regarding sexual problems. The questions and answers address issues from erectile disorder to infidelity and much more.

As you read this book, we suggest you keep a journal in order to write your responses to the "sexercises." Find the time to talk to your partner about what you are learning and ask your partner to join you in exploring your sexual needs. It can be helpful to read this book as a couple and work through the exercises together. If you come to issues that cause you to become stuck, either between you and your partner, or for you alone, consider taking this book with you, as a guide, and talking with a therapist or support person.

If you are a therapist or health-care provider, this book can be supplemental material for you to recommend to your clients. It will provide your clients with information and the tools to talk to their partners and to you.

🌿 SEXUAL HEALING

I have been with my partner for eleven years. Why do I have so much
trouble talking about sex? I talk about everything else with no problem.
I don't always get what I want in the bedroom, and I can't tell my partner what I want. What is that all about?

*This is such a common problem that we decided to write a book about
it! It's hard to pinpoint one reason, as there is a combination of reasons that make it hard to talk about sex. Were you raised not to talk
about sex, or that sex is "dirty"? Do you have sexual wounds that still
evoke shame when the subject of sex comes up? Maybe your communication skills are not what they could be. Are there some life-stage
issues you need to learn more about in order to make sexual communication more comfortable? Relationship struggles or "sore spots"
can make talking about sex much more difficult. So, as you can see,
there are numerous issues that come into play that make it hard to
talk about sex. Don't give up! It's so important to be able to talk about
sex! In order to get what we want and need, we have to communicate.
Remember that talking is only half the battle. We have to be able to
listen, as well. Read this book with your partner and work through the
exercises. Seek professional help if you feel the problem goes beyond
the scope of this book.*

🌿 🌿 🌿

As you begin the journey across the bridge, we hope that you will be
able to:

- Confront fears about expressing your sexual needs and concerns
- Examine misconceptions about sex
- Gain understanding of your sexual history
- Learn techniques to communicate about sex
- Improve your sexual relationship
- Heat up the flames of desire!

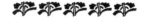

SEXERCISES

I. Consider the bridge to sexual awareness that we described earlier in this chapter. While reading the statements below, consider whether you find each statement true or false.

- I enjoy physical touch.
- I feel good about my body.
- I trust my partner.
- I am trustworthy.
- I feel good about myself.
- My family gave me positive messages about sex.
- My faith gave me positive messages about sex.
- I don't think my sex life has to reflect the media.
- I feel like I am aware of my sexual wounds.
- I have dealt with my sexual wounds (in therapy and/or with my partner).
- I understand that my partner and I have different sexual needs from each other.
- I accept that my partner may have unique likes and dislikes when it comes to sex.
- I know that life's challenges (aging, childbirth, illness, sexual disorders, emotional struggles, etc.) affect my sex life.
- My partner and I communicate effectively about sex.
- I have realistic expectations about sex.
- I know that there are many myths regarding sex.
- My partner and I have the skills to work through relationship struggles (conflict, porn, power struggles, affairs, etc).
- I am aware of what turns me on.
- I know what turns my partner on.
- I look for ways to spice up sex.
- My partner and I have regular sexy dates.
- I can easily discuss sex with my therapist.
- I can comfortably discuss sex with my health-care provider.

If you answered "false" to any of these statements, you've picked up the right book! Each of these statements will be addressed in the following chapters to help increase your awareness and give you ideas on communicating about sex. We have included in each chapter tried-and-true exercises which will spice up your sex life!

II. Establish safety rules to abide by when you are trying the exercises throughout the book (you'll find more on safety rules in chapter 6). Make your own rules so that you feel safe when you are talking to your partner. You may want to have the discussions outside of your bedroom, so your bedroom remains a safe place. Write down your rules in your journal and, if necessary, read them to each other every time you sit down to discuss sex. Consider your own safety and what you need. Each partner can share what would be safe for him or her. Do you need reassurance? When you have discussions, do you usually get to a place where you feel you are not being heard? What are triggers that might affect the way you hear your partner? Where should you have the discussions? Are interruptions a problem? Try to talk about how to end the discussion so that neither partner feels like there is unfinished business.

III. When both you and your partner are in a good place, try to think of as many sexual terms as you can! Write the terms down in your journal. Talk about what you called your body parts when you were a kid, the funny terms you have heard throughout your life, and clinical terms for body parts. Be sure and keep your sense of humor during this discussion!

IV. Begin to talk about sex on a regular basis! Try scheduling time for this conversation, focusing on one question a week, such as:

- What is a movie that had a sexual scene that really turned you on?
- Where is a great place to make love other than bed?
- What is the best erotic story you ever read?
- What music puts you "in the mood"?
- What did you think sex would be like before you actually experienced sex?

Remember to try to keep this sexercise light and fun! There will be a time to discuss heavier issues, but the goal here is to get you and your partner talking about sex. Stay away from emotionally laden questions for now. One good idea would be to write the questions down, put them in a jar, and choose one to discuss every week. That way you will always have something to discuss!

2

WHISPERS OF CHILDHOOD

Revisiting the Past

I remember feeling anxious about touch in my family. My parents
fought a lot, and I tried to stay in the background.

—Female, age 27

- What were the messages about sexuality from your childhood?
- Did you feel comfortable with touch in your childhood home?
- Were you protected from emotional and/or sexual abuse while
  growing up?
- Did your family demonstrate healthy social skills?
- When you were growing up, did you hear positive or negative mes-
  sages about your body?

In order to discuss sexual issues as adults, it's important to listen to
the whispers of childhood and the perceptions formed in early years.
Learning about the sexual self begins the moment a child is born. Family, peers, and culture all play an important role in the development
of sexuality. We may have only a dim awareness of the influence that
family environment and childhood experiences have on our sexuality.
These lessons are often subtle messages whispering to us as we attempt
to create a satisfying sexual relationship in adulthood.

We frequently struggle with our sexual interactions and wonder what forces are stirring beneath the surface. These forces are especially evident when two people, from different backgrounds, are dealing with a sexual relationship which has become strained or distant. When exploring sexuality, we need to understand our own family background and its influence.

SIX NECESSARY ELEMENTS
FOR HEALTHY SEXUAL ESTEEM

Certain critical elements, which may or may not have been present in childhood, are the foundation on which a healthy sexual esteem is built. If we are to be secure and open enough to engage in erotic and satisfying sexual activity in an intimate relationship, we must have a strong sexual sense of self. The six important elements for healthy sexual self-esteem are: appropriate touch, adequate trust, healthy body image, strong self-esteem, effective interaction skills, and appropriate boundaries.

Appropriate Touch

Appropriate touch in childhood is the first element needed to build a strong sexual foundation for adulthood. Children are touched throughout the early years due to necessity: they are fed, diapered, bathed, disciplined, comforted, toilet trained, and much more. Appropriate touch in childhood involves respectful boundaries, gentle reassurances, thoughtful gestures, and soothing expressions. However, the quality and quantity of the touch may vary greatly from home to home.

Some homes are devoid of any touch at all. People often say to us in therapy, "I know my parents loved me, but we didn't hug or kiss each other." It isn't unusual to see the following in a therapy session: a couple sitting next to each other on a small couch; one partner begins to cry while the other sits quietly, hands folded, looking straight ahead at the therapist. Comforting touch is foreign to many couples. For some, touching may not be associated with love. Then is love associated with touching?

Some homes are neglectful and a child feels invisible. The child isn't touched often and has to learn to soothe himself, even at an early age.

Chris came to therapy saying that he had had few adult sexual or emo-tional relationships. He recalled that, when he was five, a boy in his neighborhood began to bully him. The boy ran after Chris when he came outside to play, teasing and threatening him. Because Chris's parents paid little attention to him, he chose to deal with the bully on his own. He hid from this boy and tried to avoid him, but he never felt safe in his neighborhood. Chris never asked for protection from his parents because he felt he wasn't really "seen or known" by his family. As an adult, Chris explained, he had found himself with similar feelings of being invisible to his peers at work. He was uncomfortable with touch and rarely sought out intimate relationships. The emotion of fear guided him in most of his social encounters, leaving him isolated and lonely.

Some homes are filled with anxious touch. This may be due to a parent having been abused as a child, resulting in confusion about the right to touch or precisely how to touch his or her own baby, child, or teenager. At other times, this anxious touch may be associated with loss or a fear of loss that originated in the parent's own background. Some parents may be clingy or intrusive with their touch, resulting in a child who feels anxiously obligated to meet the parent's needs, at the expense of the child's own needs.

There are many homes in which there is violent touch or the threat of violence. When a household is chaotic and explosive with anger, a child learns pain and fear. The child knows that he or she needs to hide for safety or intervene to stop the violence. In these homes, touch isn't safe or soothing.

❦ SEXUAL HEALING

I have been with my partner for about a year now. Everything started out okay. He and I enjoy a lot of the same hobbies and we have friends in com-mon. But the longer we're together, we find that we have disagreements about small things. He wants to talk it out and even argue some, but I just want to avoid conflict at all costs! This has caused us to move away from each other sexually because we're not resolving problems. I came from a violent family in which my parents fought constantly. I know that I'm afraid to talk about difficult things because I don't want to get into a big fight. But I'm losing my close, fun relationship with my partner, and I hate that.

It's great that you have awareness about your fear of conflict! Often when people grow up in violent families, they don't learn how to resolve conflict, and they are afraid that all confrontation will lead to abuse. But as you've wisely pointed out, this fear of conflict has also affected you and your partner sexually.

Be sure to read chapter 6 about communication. There are ways to approach conflict and difficult subject matters without losing your cool. You and your partner will need to establish some ground rules for communicating about tough issues. Talk to your partner about your fears and about your background with conflict. Then both of you will need to practice safe communication techniques and learn to explore your differences without spiraling into explosive anger. Learning to do this will help you and your partner stay connected so that you don't feel like strangers when it comes to sex.

🌿 🌿 🌿

Some homes contain violating touch. Violating touch may be subtle or extremely overt. Sexual abuse by a parent or trusted individual leaves a child with the message that touch is dangerous and confusing.

Jennifer came to therapy to deal with her crumbling relationship. She described that she was lonely and felt rejected by her partner. He rarely wanted any physical or sexual touch from her and ridiculed Jennifer for her continued weight gain. As a child, Jennifer had been sexually molested by a significant and trusted member of her family. The molestation left her confused about touch, and she stated that the abuse and her partner's rejections caused her to feel like there was something very wrong with her. She said, "I must be a really unlovable person because this family member in my past hurt me! And I'm beginning to think that my weight gain has been a means to protect myself from male attention because it's been so painful to me."

Adequate Trust

Trust is the second crucial element for sexual well-being. Children need to know that they can turn to their parents and that their needs will be heard, understood, and handled appropriately. A child who learns that he can trust his caregivers will be able to look to others for support and understanding as he grows into a young man. Children need to be able to count on their parents to be present, both physically and emotionally.

Parents who are burdened with substance addiction or mental illness will likely be unable to perceive their child's needs and concerns. The mental disorder or substance abuse causes the parent's internal world to be chaotic and self-focused. A child in this type of home will learn to keep problems to herself or to seek answers elsewhere, realizing that she can't trust her parents to intervene effectively in her life. The child begins to take care of the needs of the parent, at the cost of getting her own needs met. She ends up in the role of parent, forfeiting her childhood. Without intervention, this role follows the child into adulthood, and she takes care of all the people around her, picking relationships with needy people who want to be taken care of by her. History then repeats itself, and she nurtures others at her own emotional expense.

Sarah, a severely depressed woman in her thirties, described in therapy that when she returns home from a day at work, she curls up in her rocking chair, blanketed by a quilt, and sinks further into her depression. Sarah often numbs herself by overusing pain medication that she has been prescribed for a past injury. Her oldest daughter, age ten, takes care of Sarah and the two younger girls until their father returns from his factory work, late at night. It was difficult for Sarah to understand the impact of her depression and medication misuse on her daughters. Sarah had little insight into her daughters' fear or sadness about their mother's condition. Sarah had trouble seeing beyond her own depression and the neglect from her own childhood. Sarah rarely touched her children, as she had little understanding of their need for affection or comfort. The three young girls learned not to trust their mother to meet their emotional or physical needs.

Due to Sarah's depression, she rarely showed affection toward her partner. In response, her partner took care of Sarah's physical needs, but was confused about how to reach Sarah emotionally. This interaction influenced the three little girls' understanding of trust, affection, and intimate relationships.

Sarah sought therapy and, after a period of treatment with heart-wrenching sessions in which she shared her guilt and shame regarding the treatment of her children, she was able to build enough strength to begin to help her girls. Sarah and the three girls began family therapy, and Sarah was able to tell them she knew that she had made some mistakes, which she was ready and willing to correct. Sarah listened quietly to her daughters, made no excuses for her past parenting, and validated their anger and other feelings. The family still had a lot of work ahead, but they were on the right path. Sarah and her partner also began couples therapy to work on their relationship.

At times, parents are emotionally and/or physically unavailable to their children because they themselves have very little insight into the importance of warmth and empathy. Empathy is the ability to understand and have insight into another's needs and feelings. Parents who demonstrate empathy are able to communicate patience and compassion to their child. If a child grows up in a family in which his parents lack empathy, he may have a difficult time as an adult trusting his partner to be empathic. Additionally, he may be unable to show adequate empathy toward his partner.

Ways of Showing Empathy to Your Child
- Speak softly
- Get down to their physical level
- Use eye contact
- Use soft and reassuring touch on the arm or shoulder
- Take a young child onto your lap
- Ask about the child's emotional state or provide words that might help them describe their emotional state
- Brainstorm ways to solve problems, giving the child the means to express strong emotions safely and appropriately
- Give an instance from your own life that was similar to the child's present problem
- Be a role model, let your child see you cry and explain your tears in an age-appropriate way (not expecting the child to "fix the hurt")
- Use problems on TV or in real life, discussing how it feels to "walk in someone else's shoes"

Healthy Body Image

A healthy body image is the third necessary element for sexual well-being. A strong body image is an important component of overall self-esteem. Some fortunate children grow up in families in which there is adequate and appropriate reassurance regarding appearance, physical changes of adolescence, and emotional or even financial assistance when physical problems arise (i.e., the need for braces, acne treatment, etc.). Many parents are able to provide compliments and assistance to their children without interfering with their child's independence, autonomy, and privacy.

However, some families may be hindrances to children in developing healthy body images. Sometimes there is teasing or criticism from parents or siblings. Many people recall being callously teased about a specific area of their body: for instance, thighs, breasts, penis, or overall weight. These memories are very difficult to erase and may lead to negativity and sensitivity about physical appearance for years afterward.

Parents play a major role in a child's body image and self-image. It's the job of the parents to tell the child she is important, point out her strengths, and let her know that life changed for the better the minute they laid eyes on her. Parents need to be involved and interested in every aspect of their child's life, while allowing some autonomy to the child at the same time. Children need to hear that parents love them, believe in them, are incredibly proud of them, and will always protect them.

We often hear that the mind is the most important sex organ in the body. If an individual's self-talk is filled with critical messages about his or her body, it's very challenging to be present, comfortable, and responsive when engaging in sexual foreplay or intercourse.

> Megan and Matt talked openly in therapy about their struggle to keep sex a priority in their busy lives. Megan admitted that she was often too tired for sex and put it off, hoping that she would feel in the mood another time. Megan also related that she was very self-conscious about her body changes after having three children. She no longer had time to exercise, and she felt too tired to do much more than go to work and take care of the kids. When talking about her childhood, Megan remembered her father saying some critical things to her about her weight when she was a teenager, and she had trouble getting those words out of her mind. She recalled that, after one of her dance recitals, her dad had said, "Megan, you're the biggest girl on stage. You need to lose some weight!" Although Matt loved Megan and felt aroused by her body, Megan's body image was fragile due to her upbringing and her perception of her physical changes with aging and childbearing.

SEXUAL HEALING

I hate to admit this—I don't feel real happy about my body and I also don't feel so great about my vagina. It's difficult for me to imagine that anyone would want anything to do with me. I haven't really looked at my genitals, but my mom used to talk about "down there" in such a negative and dirty way. This makes me very self-conscious when I'm dating someone and the physical aspect starts to heat up. Is this normal?

A lot of females and males don't feel comfortable with their genitals. It's pretty common to hear girls or women talk about feeling ugly or disgusted with their vulva area. However, this area of your body is a wonderful treasure trove of pleasure; it just needs to be explored and accepted. Every vulva looks slightly different from the next one. We have included a list of DVDs and websites that can show you more about the variations in appearance of the vulva. You'll see from these sites that everyone is different. Just as our faces don't look alike, neither do our vulvas. Don't judge yourself; no one has a perfect body.

It's a good idea to take a mirror and look at your genitals. Sit on the bed or the floor and set up a mirror so that you can touch yourself while you explore your vulva and all the various parts of your genitals. Make sure you identify your clitoris, labia majora, labia minora, vagina, and anus. Explore your body and genital area for sensitivity and pleasurable sensations. Chapter 4 contains more information about the female sexual response cycle and the important components of arousal. In the resources section, we have listed some good books and videos to help you become more familiar with and accepting of your wonderful body!

Strong Self-Esteem

Having a healthy self-esteem is the fourth element needed to become a person capable of connecting intimately with someone else. In order to feel trusting and safe in a sexual relationship, we need to respect and value ourselves. To choose a partner wisely, we must recognize our own worth and significance.

In many families, children are given sufficient love, guidance, and affection to nourish their self-worth. The parents in these families appropriately praise and support their children's efforts and accomplishments. Alternatively, other families are unable or unwilling to provide a place of warmth, safety, and growth. In these cases, the child is ignored or abused, leading to feelings of uncertainty, vulnerability, or self-hatred.

Self-esteem is also affected by the many experiences and interactions that each person has, even outside of the family. A child who is teased at school, has trouble with academic achievement, or has a difficult time fitting in with peers will find his or her self-esteem to be fragile. This tenuous self-esteem will play havoc on problem solving when it comes to emotional and sexual issues in an adult relationship. Adequate self-esteem doesn't insulate a person from the problems of life, but it does enable one to deal with the emotional difficulties in life and relationships.

Jake spoke, in therapy, of his difficulty adjusting to his current relationship. He had always been small-framed with few athletic skills. In school, Jake kept to himself on the playground and never had friends over to his house. He didn't feel he could get much attention from either parent due to their busy schedules and his many siblings needing care. When Jake began his relationship with Julie, he thought that his problems were over. He finally felt accepted and loved.

However, as the relationship progressed, Jake found that Julie was more outgoing than he had realized and that she had made many friends at her office. Julie went out with coworkers after work, and Jake thought that she seemed to be more interested in their company than in his. Jake found himself feeling some of the exact emotions that he had felt growing up—competition for attention, feeling awkward around Julie's coworkers, comparing himself to other men and feeling that he didn't measure up.

Jake's low self-esteem started to affect him sexually, as well. He felt unsure about Julie's attraction to him and so he waited for her to initiate sex. His apprehension led to a great deal of silence and many nights with each of them on opposite sides of the bed.

In therapy, Jake and Julie began to talk about their sexual and emotional distance. Julie heard Jake's long-standing feelings of low self-worth and his insecurities about her attraction to him. Julie wanted her partner to feel her love, and they began to work toward removing the wall which had unwittingly been built between them.

Effective Interaction Skills

Having effective interaction skills is the fifth element needed for healthy sexual well-being. Families with positive interaction are able to work through conflict, communicate effectively, and relate to one another rationally. There are families that have gatherings with family members, within their faith community, or within the school environment in which the interaction is pleasurable and healthy. These gatherings model for the child how to make friends, interact with others, and keep friends, even when there may be differences or disagreements.

However, there are families in which social events are filled with chaos and aggression. The child in this family learns not to invite friends over for fear of disruption or embarrassment. Children in destructive homes don't learn adequate conflict resolution skills. Additionally, children from violent and chaotic homes may become adults who fear conflict with their partner, or, on the other hand, deal with conflict in a violent manner. The inadequate problem solving will likely lead these individuals to avoid many topics, especially emotion-filled dialogues about sex.

There may be homes that are peaceful and quiet, but where no one has shown the child how to extend an invitation to a classmate for socializing. The parents in these homes usually have little understanding of socialization and may not encourage their child's interaction with others. There may also be a feeling of distance and disconnection between family members. The result is that the child in this home becomes more secluded and lacking in effective communication skills.

Jillian spoke to the therapist of her frustration with her partner, Jeremy. Jillian felt distant and cut off from Jeremy and didn't like him to touch her. Jillian explained that she was uncomfortable with Jeremy's way of interacting. She described that their friends had recently spoken to her about Jeremy's awkward monopolization of conversation at parties. Jillian agreed that Jeremy often ignored social cues in public and was equally self-absorbed at home.

Jeremy joined Jillian for couples therapy and she stated, "I think you know, Jeremy, that I'm so stressed at work. I've talked to you about this a lot, and that I need time to unwind when I get home from the office. I've asked you for this time, but you crowd me and seem oblivious to my stress. I've noticed that you do this with other people in social situations." Jeremy ap-

peared thoughtful and spoke of his own upbringing in a family that was chaotic, loud, and distracted from the real problems in the home. He recalled
his mother's constant chattering to him, while ignoring things that were
going on in Jeremy's life. After making the connection to his own family of
origin dynamics, Jeremy was willing to work on noticing social cues, and Jillian became more hopeful regarding their intimacy and sexual connection.

Effective interaction skills are important in sexual relationships because it's necessary to communicate sexual and emotional needs to one
another. Mastering social skills in childhood and adolescence teaches
partners to read body language and verbal expressions more accurately.
Childhood experiences and family dynamics may predispose a person
to strengths or vulnerabilities in the areas of communication, problem
solving, and negotiation.

Appropriate Boundaries

The sixth and final element needed for sexual well-being is boundaries, both personal and interpersonal. Boundaries are barriers that separate two things or people. Typically, there are three types of boundaries
when it comes to family interactions.[1] On one end of the spectrum is
a family that has very rigid boundaries. This family doesn't touch each
other, the family members keep to themselves, and everyone does their
own thing without much interaction. Rigid boundaries can prevent
people from having meaningful, understanding relationships with one
another. Those with rigid boundaries can be isolated and withdrawn
from others, which can be detrimental to relationships.

On the other end of the spectrum are the families with diffuse boundaries. The danger with having extremely diffuse boundaries is the risk of
enmeshment, or over-involvement in the lives of the people in the family, to the point of loss of independence. People with diffuse boundaries
have loose, undefined personal boundaries, which result in problems
defining who they are in relation to others. People with diffuse boundaries often are clingy, needy, and dependent on others.

Healthy boundaries are called clear boundaries, and they allow a child
to come into the arms of the family to get his needs met, but also to step
outside the family to gain independence. This boundary system allows a
person to go easily between moving away from and moving back into the
family.

Appropriate boundaries play a vital part in sexual behavior and relationships. If a family exhibits poor or loose sexual boundaries, the child in this family may begin to believe that his body isn't his own. Subsequently, as this child develops, he may have sexual experiences that are actually unwanted or that cross personal boundaries or values. The child may find himself seeking sexual experiences in order to be assured of self-worth, or he may come to feel that sex is "expected." If the sexual boundaries are rigid and sexual messages are silent, the child may grow up to avoid sexual intimacy, see sex as wrong, or not have an age-appropriate understanding of sex.

What are "red flags" that adult behavior is crossing a child's sexual boundaries?

- Flirting with a child or kissing inappropriately
- Making lewd comments or jokes
- Letting a child see an adult "ogling" or being sexually disrespectful of another person
- Telling a child that sex and body parts are dirty, nasty, or stinky, or using other derogatory descriptions of them
- Allowing a child to view provocative material in magazines, on TV, or on the computer
- Complimenting a child or teen on explicitly private body areas (i.e., penis size, breast size or appearance, rear)
- Discussing private sexual concerns or experiences with a child that pertain to the adults in his or her world
- Being sexually intimate with a child
- After the age of four or five, allowing the child to see an adult naked or bathing
- Not allowing the child privacy
- Washing a child's genitals after about the age of four or five
- Touching inappropriately

SEXUAL HEALING

When I think about the six necessary elements for sexual well-being, I have deficits in every one! In my childhood, one of my male cousins sexually molested me. I'm a male and this molestation has been a source of deep shame all of my life. As a kid, when I told my mom about the mo-lestation, she sort of brushed it off. She told me not to hang out with my cousin any more, but we never talked about it again. Also, I have always compared myself to other guys or to pictures in magazines and I'm never satisfied with my looks. My self-esteem is pretty low! I have never felt confident with my social skills so I don't like going out with my partner and her friends. As you can imagine, this is all taking its toll on our rela-tionship and sex life. I don't feel confident and I have a lot of shame!

Sometimes it's difficult to look deeply at the effects of childhood, but you're making progress in examining these crucial elements. Chapter 3 will go into more depth about sexual abuse and its effects on sexuality, but you are right to begin to explore what effect this molestation had on your feelings about touch, boundaries, and trust. Be sure to talk to your partner about all of these areas. It would be helpful to do this in therapy, where you can have some guidance in understanding the path to healing from abuse. It's likely that your partner doesn't fully understand your reluctance to engage sexually or even socially. It will be helpful to open up to her about your fears, your low self-esteem, and your body image issues.

MESSAGES FROM OTHERS ABOUT SEX

In addition to the six elements from childhood that influence sexuality, verbal and nonverbal messages from family, peers, the media, culture, and the person's faith community also affect each individual. Mom, dad, siblings, classmates, teachers, preachers, relatives, dating partners, mov-ies, song lyrics, and total strangers express messages about sexuality, both knowingly and unknowingly. These messages come from direct verbal communication and from subtle nonverbal gestures or tone of voice. The messages may be positive, negative, unrealistic, or even heavy silences.

Positive Messages about Sexuality

The positive messages regarding sexuality during childhood include age-appropriate information, respectful answers to questions about sex, and honest attempts to seek answers when there is confusion or when troubling behavior needs to be addressed. Positive sexual messages also include the teaching that a healthy, respectful sexual relationship is essential for couples. One loving response to childhood and adolescent sexual curiosity is to provide accurate books and other resources that teach appropriate and positive messages about sexuality, body image, and realistic expectations. Additionally, an appropriate response to adolescent sexual exploration is to provide information about sexually transmitted infections and the means by which to prevent pregnancy.

Resources to Help Kids and Teens Learn about Sexuality

- Carroll, Janell L. *The Day Aunt Flo Comes to Visit: An Honest Conversation about Getting Your Period*
- Haffner, Debra W. *From Diapers to Dating: A Parent's Guide to Raising Sexually Healthy Children*
- Harris, Robie H., and Michael Emberly. *It's NOT the Stork! A Book about Girls, Boys, Babies, Bodies, Families and Friends*
- Levin, Diane E., and Jean Kilbourne. *So Sexy So Soon: The New Sexualized Childhood and What Parents Can Do to Protect Their Kids*
- Levkoff, Logan. *Third Base Ain't What It Used to Be: What Your Kids Are Learning about Sex and How to Teach Them to Become Sexually Healthy Adults*
- Libby, Roger W. *The Naked Truth about Sex: A Guide to Intelligent Sexual Choices for Teenagers and Twentysomethings*
- Miron, Amy G., and Charles D. Miron. *How to Talk to Teens about Love, Relationships, and S-E-X: A Guide for Parents*
- Pardes, Bronwen. *Doing It Right: Making Smart, Safe, and Satisfying Choices about Sex*
- Redd, Nancy Amanda. *Body Drama: Real Girls, Real Bodies, Real Issues, Real Answers*
- Schoen, Mark. *Bellybuttons Are Navels*
- www.goaskalice.columbia.edu
- www.iwannaknow.org
- www.kidshealth.org/teen
- www.oprah.com/article/oprahshow/20090326-tows-talking-to-kids-about-sex-handbook
- www.scarleteen.com
- www.teenwire.com

Negative Messages about Sexuality

Negative messages related to sexuality include derogatory, insulting, and demeaning responses to questions or situations. Parents may give children very negative views about the body, genitals, or intercourse. For example, a young male teen might be discovered masturbating or looking at sexually explicit material. A reasoned reaction to this situation is required so that the teenager doesn't feel shamed or embarrassed about his curiosity and normal male responses. Another example of negative communication regarding sexuality would be a mother imparting private information to her daughter or son about her own lack of sexual desire for her partner. The child, in this situation, is burdened with information about a private matter. These negative messages will be carried into adulthood and can be played out in direct or indirect behaviors in a sexual relationship.

 SEXUAL HEALING

My partner really wants me to wear sexy lingerie to bed, but I'm so reluctant to do this! I grew up knowing that my dad looked at a lot of porn and my mom hated it! She'd scream at my dad about it sometimes, and she also would tell me that men are just animals and all they want is sex! My partner is a pretty normal guy, I think, but I find myself hearing my mom's voice in my head and worry that my partner will eventually want something else from me sexually that I'll find perverted. I guess I'm afraid to indulge this request, and I know I don't look anything like the girls in lingerie catalogs!

It IS difficult to get those voices from the past to be silent sometimes! Your partner sounds like most guys who want to spice things up in the bedroom or even act out a fantasy of his own. Your mother's words are powerful, and it sounds like your dad had some real issues with porn. But even if this isn't the issue in your relationship, be sure to talk to your partner about your fears and discomfort. Trust him to understand the pressure that you feel to have the "perfect" body and that you will feel a bit self-conscious at first. Also explore with your partner your fear that this request will lead to other desires or fantasies of his and that you're afraid you won't feel comfortable with them. Allow your partner to know these important aspects of your sexual self.

❈ ❈ ❈

Unrealistic Messages about Sexuality

The media provides many unrealistic messages about sexuality and relationships. There are few movies or soap operas in which the main characters are dealing with an aging body, the need for lubrication, or erectile dysfunction. Rarely is there a film in which a couple is depicted in a long-term relationship, solving conflicts with respect, and still being affectionate with one another. It is more common to see affairs and steamy scenes with beautiful actors in magnificent bedrooms, with no children knocking at the door!

Males in our society are especially vulnerable to the unrealistic images and stories about male sexuality. Frequently the message given to a man is that he will be ready for sex at a moment's notice, that his erection will always be hard enough, and that he will have the skills and techniques to bring a woman to amazing orgasms. These expectations are often perpetuated by porn, by teenagers' stories of their sexual exploits, and by long-held beliefs in our society of what constitutes being a "real man." These messages put a great deal of pressure on a man, especially as he ages.

Girls and women in our society also have many demands on them to resemble the females portrayed in magazines and film. Teenagers and even adult women often talk about their struggle to lose weight or accept their body or face when they feel that they aren't living up to an expectation of what is acceptable. If a woman's perception is that she isn't sexy enough or thin enough or voluptuous enough, she will likely have a difficult time being present in sexual situations. Often a woman emphasizes the importance of being the object of her partner's desire, rather than appreciating and celebrating her body, its sexual responses, and her own uniqueness.

Silences about Sexuality

A person's background might include a home in which there was a great deal of silence among family members and secrets regarding sexuality. Some women report, "My mom told me nothing about menstruation. I was shocked and embarrassed the first time it happened!" A young man might be confused about female anatomy and have no one in whom to confide. There may be a sense of secrecy regarding some aspect of the family's background that relates to sexuality. For example, some families don't discuss a past of sexual abuse, rape, abortion, unplanned pregnancy, or a child who was given up for adoption.

 ## SEXUAL HEALING

My mom didn't want to acknowledge that I was sexually active in my late teens so I went with a friend to a clinic to be put on birth control. I have now been sexually involved with my partner for about three years, and we have decided to live together. Upon hearing that we will be moving in together, my mother finally sat me down and told me to be careful about the possibility of unwanted pregnancy. I assured my mom that I'd been dealing with this issue responsibly for the past five years! She then blurts out that she got pregnant in her teens and gave up a son for adoption. I had no idea! This explains a lot of things about my mother's relationship with me and her distance from her own family. I wish she'd been able to deal with this when it happened, like getting therapy. And I wish she and I had been able to talk more openly all these years!

It's not uncommon for people to hold on to secrets, especially those that are sexual in nature. It helps to be able to talk with parents about their own childhood or adolescence when the time is right. It can shed light on family dynamics and on your own struggles with sexuality or body image. This can be a long journey as you share this with your mother, and therapy may certainly help.

✿ ✿ ✿

We often assume that our partner has similar views about sex or about his or her body when, in fact, the experiences may differ dramatically. Many of us have areas in our lives about which we are silent or ashamed. It's not unusual to find that, when couples in therapy begin sharing on a deeper level, they will say to one another, "I never knew that about you until now!"

Beth and Ben entered therapy in order to address their desire discrepancy. Ben felt that his desire had diminished in the past two years of their relationship, while Beth continued to feel as interested in sex as she was when they were first together. Ben stated that he felt ashamed of his low desire because most of his male friends complained about the fact that they wanted more sex than their partners did. Ben thought there was something wrong with him, and Beth was beginning to feel unattractive to Ben because he moved away from her when she wanted to be sexual.

Ben and Beth grew up with very different backgrounds. Beth's family was loving and affectionate, and she felt safe to go to her parents with her problems and needs. Ben's mother raised him without his father, and she often allowed other men into her life who were abusive toward her and Ben. Ben recalled hearing his mother called names and being thrown against the bedroom wall. It was common to hear these men, usually drunk, demanding sex from Ben's mother.

As Ben recalled his upbringing, it became clear to him that he feared his own sexual urges. Ben remembered the men who degraded his mother. The verbal abuse toward Ben's mother was often sexual in nature. Ben described to Beth that his own sexual desires had become confusing over the years because he found himself remembering his mother's abuse.

Beth reacted with sadness for Ben's painful memories and experiences, but she also was grateful that she finally understood his struggles. She explained, "I never knew that the abuse toward your mother was so horrific and I also didn't realize how sexual it was! I now understand, Ben, how difficult it must be for you to experience our affection, touching, and sexuality without the overlap of memories from your childhood. Thank you for telling me!"

What do these overt and covert messages teach? We may be only vaguely aware of the influence that others have had. It's helpful for us to search the recesses of our minds for the teachings from childhood regarding assumptions, unrealistic expectations, or negative thoughts about sex.

Our childhoods whisper to us in many ways . . . sometimes murmuring quietly and sometimes screaming at the top of their lungs! Although there are both positive and painful aspects to what we faced as children, it's necessary to remember that our childhood experiences made us who we are—even the negative, painful events in our lives. We couldn't be who we are without them. We need to celebrate who we are, both the positive and the negative. Don't let the whispers of childhood drown out the conversations of adulthood. Know that we can be stronger people because of what we experienced, and not victims of our past. If you have difficulty dealing with the past, seek a therapist to help you. Chapter 10 in this book gives you tips for finding a good therapist.

MOVING ACROSS THE BRIDGE

Touch, trust, body image, self-esteem, interaction skills, and appropriate boundaries are all essential ingredients to healthy adult sexuality. Even without your being consciously aware of these six elements, they have each made their mark on your sexual self-esteem. Additionally, sexual messages—positive, negative, unrealistic, or silent—taught you about your sexuality and your body. Your childhood whispers many important clues about the ways in which you currently express your sexual needs.

❧❧❧❧❧

SEXERCISES

I. The experiences you had in childhood and adolescence are important in the development of your sexual self. Each of the six necessary elements has been described in the chapter. Now each will be listed with questions for you to consider. Using your journal, write answers to the following questions and then talk with your partner about whatever you feel comfortable sharing.

- *Touch*: How was I touched in my home? Was touch comforting or disturbing? Did I feel safe with my parents, siblings, and other family members? Did anyone touch me without my permission? Was I abused physically or sexually?
- *Trust*: Could I trust my parents to protect me? Could I trust my family to care for me, listen to me, and pay attention to my needs? Did I feel empathy in my home?
- *Body Image*: How did I feel about my body when I was growing up? Did others respect my privacy? Did I get realistic compliments from family and friends? Did anyone degrade, humiliate, or criticize my body and me?

- *Self-Esteem*: Did I like myself growing up? Did others in my family and peer group want to be with me and seem to appreciate me? Did I succeed at things while growing up (in school, at home, in my faith community, or with peers)? Did I feel adequate, well-liked, appreciated, and noticed?
- *Effective Interaction Skills*: Did I make friends easily? Did I keep my friends for long periods of time? Was I terribly shy or withdrawn? Did my family resolve conflicts effectively? Was I encouraged to socialize? Was my family chaotic or aggressive?
- *Appropriate Boundaries*: What boundaries were crossed by my family? How was I told about sex? Did my family have flimsy boundaries? Were family boundaries too rigid? How did the boundaries in my family affect my ability to define myself in adolescence? Did I see displays of appropriate affection in my family?

II. How does each of the following areas influence your current relationship? Write about your feelings and thoughts in your journal and talk with your partner about what you learn.

- How do I feel about *touch* in this current relationship? What would I like to change regarding touch?
- Do I *trust* myself and do I trust my partner? What are the areas of distrust?
- Do I feel good about my *body image* and can I accept compliments from my partner? How does my body image affect my physical, emotional, and sexual relationship?
- Do I feel adequate in my relationship? Is my *self-esteem* too low and does this interfere with my ability to be affectionate or to accept affection? What are some reasons that my self-esteem is low?
- How are my *interaction skills*? How is my childhood affecting my ability to communicate my sexual needs to my partner?
- What are my *boundaries* in my current relationship? What are the sexual messages I received that affect the way I perceive sex and my genitals?

III. Look back at old family photographs and examine facial expressions, family member placement, and touch as depicted in these pictures.

Write in your journal about what you learn as you look back at old photographs. Did your family appear close? Are there only a few pictures? Did your family look tense, happy, fun-loving, relaxed, distant?

IV. Using your journal, describe any messages that you received, while growing up, about sex, anatomy, or gender from each of the following:

Parents
Siblings
Other Family Members
Peers
Teachings from Faith Community
Media
Teachers

If you feel comfortable, share these messages with your partner.

V. As we grow up, we have influences from many sources. Often we take these messages with us in the form of self-talk. For three days, write down any negative self-talk that you find yourself having. For example, "I hate my gut!" "My legs are so flabby!" "My partner's an idiot!" or "My partner's a nag."

To the side of each negative thought, write down a positive or neutral alternative thought.

For instance, "I hate my gut!" can be changed to "My stomach is bigger than I'd like, but I am forty-three years old, and I'm proud of myself for doing crunches this morning." Or, "My partner's an idiot!" can be changed to "My partner helped me unload the dishwasher yesterday and he's a great dad."

3

ECHOES OF SEXUAL SECRETS

Healing the Wounds

I have so much shame from my past. I've kept a lot of secrets, but I finally feel that I need to talk about things with my partner.

—Male, age 46

- Are you struggling with the sexual effects of childhood abuse?
- Has rape affected your sexual relationship with your partner?
- Are you a gay, lesbian, bisexual, or transgender individual who has suffered prejudice and/or discrimination?
- Does masturbation bring up feelings of shame for you?

In the last chapter, we discussed different ways that sexual perceptions are developed. A person's sexual experience is multifaceted, shaped by culture, upbringing, personality characteristics, and biological framework.

What happens when our perceptions become distorted by sexual wounds? Sexual wounds leave scars on men and women that can affect sexuality and many other areas of life. Shame and secrets become part of one's perception of sex. Shame may prevent us from expressing our true sexual selves when it comes to issues such as sexual abuse, rape, sexual orientation, and masturbation. These subjects are hard to deal with on our own, inside ourselves, let alone communicate to others! If we can learn to accept who we are with all our experiences, realize we can't change certain aspects of our lives, and work through past trauma, then it becomes easier to discuss the issues in the context of our relationships. It is a rare person who goes through life with no incidence of sexual shame. We have all been exposed to sexual wounds, which might have been caused by parents who wouldn't talk about sex, shaming religious ideas, abstinence-only educational programs, or inadequate sexual boundaries.

How do sexual wounds affect sexuality during childhood and adulthood? Sexual wounds can cause deep feelings of shame and difficulty expressing one's sexuality. This chapter is meant to be informative and provide suggestions, but it shouldn't substitute for professional help. It's a necessary discussion of how our sexual beliefs can become distorted, but it can provide only a small amount of information for a very difficult and important topic. Chapter 10 gives suggestions for finding a qualified therapist who can help with feelings and insights, while providing the emotional support necessary to begin to heal from sexual wounds.

If you have sexual wounds, chances are that you are struggling with the aftermath. We recommend that you seek professional help.

SEXUAL ABUSE

One type of sexual wound can be sexual abuse as a child and/or being sexually demeaned or harassed. It's difficult to know the true prevalence of child sexual abuse because this type of abuse is usually underreported. Commonly cited studies in community samples report that approximately 33 percent of girls under the age of eighteen and 5–10 percent of boys the same age are victims of sexual abuse.[1] Wendy Maltz, in her book, *The Sexual Healing Journey*, describes abuse as the following: "Sexual abuse occurs whenever one person dominates and exploits another by means of sexual activity or suggestion."[2] Abuse can be anywhere along a continuum of experiences, from lewd remarks, to being fondled once, to molestation, to rape. Family members, family friends, or even strangers could be perpetrators.

> Jane came to therapy very distraught. She said that she had been in and out of relationships that typically began as sexual encounters. Jane said

that since her last breakup, she had started "sleeping around." After a few therapy sessions, Jane hesitantly revealed that a "family friend" had sexually abused her from the time she was six until she was fifteen years old. Jane struggled with the shame of finally revealing the secret and the feeling that she was "damaged goods." She began to realize in therapy that the abuse wasn't her fault, even though the man who abused her told her that it *was* her fault for wearing "skimpy" clothing when he was around. He threatened Jane that, if she told anyone, they would think bad things about her. She was also able to come to terms with the fact that she didn't have to have sex with someone to feel cared for and loved. It was a long, difficult journey for Jane, but one that helped her begin to learn healthy sexual behavior and improve her feelings of self-worth. By finally revealing her secret, Jane was able to begin to empower herself and take the power away from her abuser.

Childhood sexual abuse interrupts the normal development of trust, a sense of safety, healthy sexuality, and comfort. A survivor is likely to experience feelings of loss, grief, shame, fear, distrust, anger, sadness, and low self-esteem. The memories and emotional consequences can lead to flashbacks, substance abuse, depression, self-destructive behavior, and relationship problems. These are symptoms that interfere with self-esteem and sexual comfort so it is imperative that a survivor seek appropriate therapy.

Confusion and Shame Associated with Sexual Abuse

Uncertainty and confusion about sex become problems for survivors. Feelings of confusion are common because the time when sexual abuse was occurring may have been the only time the person received any affection or attention. Additionally, if a parent was the perpetrator, the other parent may have actually been jealous or blaming. Furthermore, there is often a sense of shame because the survivor may feel that their body betrayed them, allowing for pleasurable sensations and even orgasm during the abuse.

The bottom line is that the survivor did nothing to cause the abuse and could not *ever* have prevented it. The perpetrator was only concerned with getting his or her own needs met. Even if the survivor was bribed, received gifts, received certain privileges, or escaped punishment, it is not the survivor's fault and he or she could not have stopped the abuse. The survivor was coerced and the abuser was more powerful than the survivor was.

What about Men Who Have Been Sexually Abused?

As with females, males in our society can be sexually abused as children, causing many aftereffects. Mike Lew points out in his helpful book for male survivors, *Victims No Longer*, that "not only does our perception of men (and of victimization) set a context for abuse, it provides a backdrop for our perception of the male survivor."[3] Males in our culture are expected to be strong and able to protect themselves and, if victimized, be able to deal with the assault in a macho manner. Lew explains that boys are usually taught the male problem-solving approach, which is to avenge the hurt and then forget about the abuse or problem. He states that, once abuse has occurred, a male survivor may feel that he has to be in control of his feelings of anger, fear, and confusion; if he can't control these emotions, he may feel that he has failed as a man.

Ethan came to therapy saying that he had been depressed and struggling with low sexual desire. The therapist learned that a male teacher had sexually abused Ethan as a child. Ethan stated that he was engaged but not sure he could go through with the marriage. He told the therapist that he didn't feel like "much of a man," and that he sees himself as "weak." He wondered if he really "wanted" the abuse because he wasn't able to stop the teacher from abusing him. After participating in therapy, Ethan was able to understand that children cannot stop abuse, and that the abuse didn't make him less of a man. Ethan was on the road to finding his sexual self and realizing his identity as a male. He and his fiancée worked in therapy together to understand the sexual abuse and its impact on their emotional and sexual life.

Peter Dimock conducted a study investigating the characteristics of adult males who were sexually abused as children, finding three common characteristics: sexual compulsiveness, masculine identity confusion, and relationship dysfunction.[4] The study defined sexual compulsiveness as addictive behavior, in which the male survivor exhibited behaviors such as excessive masturbation, having multiple sexual partners, and performing sexual acts in public places. The survivors reported feeling remorse and shame after engaging in these behaviors. Confusion about masculinity presented in two ways in Dimock's study: confusion about sexual orientation and confusion regarding male gender roles. Confusion about sexual orientation ranged from same-sex attraction to heterosexual men who had questions about their orientation and related these questions directly to the abuse. Additionally, the male survivors indicated feelings of failure as males for being vulnerable and weak. Finally, all of the men in this study who were in relationships were having difficulty in them. They all had difficulty establishing trusting, steady relationships. Many experienced relationships that would be intense for a period and then they would withdraw. The men tended to vacillate back and forth between these states.

How Does Sexual Abuse Affect Sex?

There are many ways that sexual abuse may affect a person's sexual self. In the book *Guide to Getting It On*, Paul Joannides explains that when a woman who has been sexually abused receives normal sexual stimulation that is arousing, the woman may be confused and see it as danger instead of a pleasurable experience.[5] The person can become ready for "fight or flight" instead of the excitement that someone who has not been sexually abused might feel. More than likely, this is a protective measure that the body uses, which interferes with sexual encounters.

There are specific triggers that may bring up the past trauma, and these triggers are different for each person, such as a look, the weight of someone's body, the feel of a penis, the smell of cologne, or the tug at a nipple. It's important that a survivor has an understanding partner who knows what was endured. Using a signal or a certain word when triggered may be a helpful way for a survivor to give his or her partner a heads-up that there is a problem.

Possible Symptoms of Sexual Abuse
- Flashbacks and/or nightmares
- Hypervigilance (an abnormally heightened awareness of the environment)
- Anger
- Shame and/or guilt
- Promiscuity

- Avoiding relationships and sex
- Fear
- Eating problems
- Problems with sexual desire and arousal
- Problems with orgasm
- Substance abuse
- Emotional numbing
- Dissociating (This is a defense mechanism that some people use to deal with trauma. An example is a child who fixates on TV during sexual abuse in an effort not to acknowledge or feel what's going on. Some survivors continue to dissociate, even years after the abuse. Some describe it as a sense of "checking out" or not being "present").
- Depression and/or anxiety

 SEXUAL HEALING

I'm in a relationship with someone who has been sexually abused. I know that my partner is trying to do what is needed to heal, seeking therapy and a support group. I feel so helpless! I feel ashamed because sometimes I get so impatient. I don't blame my partner, but I'm mad as hell that the person who caused this still continues to hold us hostage! What can I do to help my partner and myself?

It's critical for the two of you to keep the lines of communication open. This will allow safety and freedom to share important information about triggers, emotions, sexual needs, and ways to be helpful to each other. Remember, sexual abuse usually means harboring secrets, so discussing and communicating can be an antidote, making your relationship very different from the hush-hush incidence of abuse.

As the partner of an abuse survivor, be sure that you are taking care of yourself and your own needs. This does not mean ignoring your partner; it means taking care of yourself first. It's kind of like the steward's instruction on an airplane when he tells you to give oxygen to yourself before seeing to your child if the cabin pressure decreases. You can't be supportive to another person if you're struggling for breath yourself. Do things you enjoy doing and be sure you have a support system in place that you can depend on when life gets tough. It's normal for you to have emotions such as impatience. You may feel helpless that you can't take all the pain away from your partner. You may also feel angry at the abuser. Be cautious, you may want to rescue your partner, sometimes at the expense of your own needs and feelings. The reality is that you can't fix this and your partner has to work through some of this alone, but it's great to be supportive.

So, What about the Partner of the Survivor?

When one person in a relationship has experienced sexual abuse, there has to be a balance in dealing with the issues that ensue. Fault and blame need to be thrown out of the picture; they are simply not helpful. Each person in the relationship has individual needs and feelings and both must be addressed. The survivor has to be allowed to take the lead in the relationship due to the trauma. One of the characteristics of abuse is the loss of choice and being forced to do something that is not desired; therefore, it's healthy to have some psychological and physical control in healing.

A partner of a survivor needs to learn as much as possible about sexual trauma. It's important to know that emotions are going to run high at times and the abuse effects will surface at different times throughout the relationship. There will be behaviors that may not always be easy to understand and may seem directed at the partner, but are actually meant for the perpetrator.

According to Eliana Gil in her book, *Outgrowing the Pain*, the survivor may often behave in a way to try to recreate abuse because he or she may feel as though they don't deserve a loving partner.[6] Gil elaborates by saying that the survivor may fall back on what she or he knows is familiar, instead of the unknown. Further, a lot of anxiety surrounds the unfamiliar.

Another reason for this phenomenon is that the survivor may recreate the abusive situation in an attempt to come to terms with the abuse and to "make it stop." This is not because the survivor wants to re-experience the trauma, but because the re-creation becomes a coping mechanism for dealing with the abuse. The person who was abused may unconsciously hope to change "history" if the trauma is re-created and he or she is able to finally make it stop; this is done in an effort to empower him- or herself. Unfortunately, it rarely works that way.

If you are the partner of a survivor of sexual abuse and find yourself drawn into chaos in your relationship, this may actually be tapping into a childhood dynamic with which you are familiar. For example, you may have had a childhood with turbulence and chaos. If the relationship is draining your emotional resources, this is a good time to seek individual or couples therapy.

How Do We Heal from Abuse?

Many factors determine how a man or a woman deals with abuse. Every survivor has his or her own unique story. For example, a person who was sexually abused may have had to keep secrets, never telling for fear of what others might think, or for fear of being hurt. Another person may have been abused, the trauma revealed in some way, and the family did what was needed to protect the survivor: therapy, legal involvement, and support. These two people will deal with the abuse in very different ways. Keep in mind that neither way of handling the secrets and shame is wrong; they were two very different situations. Other factors that determine how someone reacts to abuse include whether the survivor was believed or not, if he or she told, the survivor's personality traits, how others reacted to the trauma, the severity of the trauma, the survivor's own self-esteem, the length of time it lasted, who the abuser was in the survivor's life, and how old the survivor was at the time. Again, it is important to seek help from a qualified therapist who can consider all these things and help find appropriate healing.

In the book, *The Courage to Heal*, Ellen Bass and Laura Davis state that the best sign of healing is that the shame becomes less.[7] The most effective way to begin dealing with the shame is to talk about the abuse. Wendy Maltz suggests several reasons that a survivor might remain silent, such as embarrassment about the abuse, not wanting to be seen as a victim, being seen as less of a man/woman, losing social standing, being told not to tell, and being afraid of the reaction others might have toward them.[8] Secrets keep us from being able to move forward. Remember the old adage, "We're as sick as our secrets." Whether we acknowledge the secrets or not, they are always there. If we push them away, they tend to come out "sideways," such as in the form of depression, anxiety, shame, or anger that have no apparent cause.

 ## SEXUAL HEALING

My lesbian partner and I are struggling in our sexual relationship. I have been unable to stay present with her when we are intensely sexual because I have flashbacks to my sexual abuse as a child. My parents were not open about sex, but they didn't help me have much privacy in a home with four brothers. I had to share a bathroom with my brothers, as we were poor and had a small house. I also remember that my parents left me with my siblings for long hours in the summer when my parents worked in the nearby town. It was during one particular summer that my oldest brother sexually abused me while my parents were away at work. I never came right out and told my parents, but I showed a lot of fear and asked them not to leave me alone with my brothers again. They made other arrangements for me, but never talked to me about my fears. Now the memories of my brother's actions are coming back to me, and I wish that I'd been able to talk to my folks about it all when I was a child.

Your experience with flashbacks related to sexual abuse is something about which many survivors talk. The silence after abuse is a common occurrence. You're right, it would have been helpful to have had your parents talk with you and protect you when you were a child. The silence that you experienced in your home sometimes teaches an unfortunate lesson—be quiet and things will just go away. However, staying quiet about what happened to you and about the flashbacks will not serve you well. We encourage you to read about how to "ground" yourself during sex so that you can be "anchored" in the present and can find reassurance from your partner. In the resources section of this book, you can find books and DVDs that will help you learn about "anchoring" techniques and relearning touch. We also have included a "grounding" exercise in the sexercises at the end of this chapter.

Communication is key to healing from sexual wounds. Sexual abuse is a secret that carries a great deal of shame and will often lie trapped in the survivor's psyche. Being able to discuss the trauma frees the survivor from the stifling grasp of the perpetrator. The secret no longer has any power over the abused. Finally communicating moves the victim to the status of "survivor."

Trust needs to be established through communication between loving partners. If there is no safe partner, it's best to find a good friend who is trustworthy, as well as a therapist who is experienced in the treatment of sexual abuse. When talking about sexual abuse, it's critical to have a safety net. Refer to chapter 6 for tips on communicating and establishing a safe harbor to discuss this sensitive issue.

ADULT RAPE

What defines rape? Rape is sex that is not consensual, whether it's oral, anal, or vaginal intercourse. It can be a violent act based on fear, or one in which a person isn't in the frame of mind to make a clear decision, such as when drugs or alcohol is involved. Rape is a sexual wound that causes shame for men and women. Some survivors of rape blame themselves, thinking there is something they could have done to prevent the incident. This is not the case. Rape is about control for the perpetrator and has nothing to do with the survivor's sexuality. Rape is rape, and it's a violation of a person's body. Because of the degree of shame involved, many rapes go unreported, and the survivor lives life with a secret and no support. We know that only one in five rapes is ever reported, so out of the five people, only one person is getting the help and support he or she needs. The number of unreported rapes climbs even higher for same-sex rape.

Have You Been Raped?

Consider these questions:

• Were you not able to agree to consensual sex because you were under the influence of drugs or alcohol?

- Did someone give you drugs without your knowledge and then force you to have sex?
- Did you say "no" to sex and were forced to have sex anyway?
- Did someone coerce you into sex using fear tactics or threats?
- Did you decide in the midst of sexual activity that you didn't want to continue, but were forced to go on with it?

If you are a rape victim, seek help. There are resources out there to help you, whether it was last week or ten years ago.

If you were raped, here are some resources:
- www.med.unc.edu/alcohol/prevention/rape
- www.NSVRC.org
- www.rainn.org
- www.rapeis.org
- Local hospital emergency room
- Local police station

Date Rape

Statistics show that most rape victims know the person who raped them. Whether the person knew the perpetrator of rape or not, the emotions and reactions are consistent. There are many ways rape might happen other than violently forcing a person to have sex. Date rape drugs, coercion, or threats are generally more common in date or acquaintance rape than sheer force. The bottom line is that rape is rape, no matter what method the rapist chooses to use and no matter how well the victim knows the perpetrator. It is still sexual assault with devastating consequences.

Post-Traumatic Stress Disorder

Often, according to Judith Herman, post-traumatic stress disorder is diagnosed when a person has been sexually abused as a child or an adult.[9] Post-traumatic stress disorder can be diagnosed if a person has experienced or witnessed a traumatic event which involved serious injury or threat to a person's physical being. The trauma results in intense emotions and reactions. Post-traumatic stress disorder is treatable, but a professional who is familiar with treating trauma is needed.

Symptoms That May Occur with Post-Traumatic Stress Disorder (Diagnostic and Statistical Manual of Mental Disorders-IV-TR):[10]
- Flashbacks or nightmares
- Distress caused by any event that is similar to the original trauma
- Avoidance of any situation that is similar to the trauma
- No memory of important details of the trauma
- Lack of interest in activities
- Sense of detachment from others
- Restricted range of emotions or feelings
- No sense of a future
- Sleep problems
- Irritability and anger
- Startles easily
- Hypervigilance (very aware of one's surroundings)

If you struggle with some of these symptoms and have witnessed or experienced trauma, check with a health-care or mental health provider.

 SEXUAL HEALING

Several years ago, a person I went out on one date with raped me. It was a violent attack, and I am having problems with nightmares and flashbacks. I'm also on edge most of the time and I jump when someone touches me. I'm angry for no reason, I push my partner away, and nothing seems fun anymore. I don't know what's wrong with me!

The response you are describing sounds like post-traumatic stress disorder, and you should see a psychologist who can diagnose and treat the disorder. When a person experiences trauma, the body goes into a mode of protection. The problem is that, long after the danger is gone, your mind and your nervous system continue to act as if the threat is still there. Sex and pleasure are not on the priority list; your body is registering only the act of survival. You might feel as though you are constantly on guard, so in this state of anxiety, any pleasure falls by the wayside. The next section talks about our sexual responses to trauma.

Avoidant and Compulsive Sexual Behavior

When a person has suffered sexual wounds, there may be problems that occur with normal sexual responses; these reactions tend to vary. Dr. Stephanie Buehler suggests that those who suffered childhood sexual abuse tend to have incidences of both hypersexual behaviors and avoidant behaviors surrounding sexual activity, although the literature to date fails to explain what determines each type of response.[11]

With any type of traumatic sexual experience, there are different ways of reacting, which may occur weeks, months, or even years after the trauma happened. One type of response is low desire or a tendency to be disgusted or scared of sex, a reaction that is similar to the urge to "flee" from a traumatic sexual incident. Another type of response is to "check out" or dissociate during sex. This is when a person thinks about the shopping list or watches TV during sex, instead of being engaged with his or her partner. Some sexual assault survivors have sex compulsively in an attempt to gain control over sex, when in reality, sex becomes out of control.

Buehler tells us that, for females who are sexually abused as children, some of the hormones that are associated with the stress response are elevated with the incidence of repeated sexual abuse and can increase sexual behavior. This is because the hormones may bring on the onset of early puberty, which can lead to early sexual activity. Buehler suggests that a physician needs to screen for childhood sexual abuse and refer appropriately.

INTERNALIZED SHAME FOR GLBT PERSONS

Why address shame for gay, lesbian, bisexual, and transgender (GLBT) persons in this section of the book about sexual wounds? Societal stigma and discrimination contribute to internalized experiences of shame for people who are gay, lesbian, bisexual, and transgender. It wasn't until

1986 that homosexuality was completely removed from the *Diagnostic and Statistical Manual*, which diagnoses mental illness and disorders in the field of psychology and psychiatry. The American Psychological Association states that psychologists have determined that the kind of prejudice, violence, and discrimination that the GLBT population suffers from has detrimental psychological effects.[12] We know that GLBT persons often experience verbal harassment or abuse and they have been discriminated against in housing and employment, unless protected by laws that are enforced.

"Coming out" is the process of telling others about same-sex attractions or identifying as a transgender person. Research indicates that the coming out process is important for psychological well-being and integrating sexual orientation into the person's life. Shame can prevent this disclosure, leaving the person feeling unable to share his or her life with the people around them, as well as unable to receive the support of others. Studies have shown that GLBT persons can have good, stable relationships that are remarkably similar to those of heterosexual married couples.

Joe Kort describes the way our society deals with those of different sexual orientations as "sexual trauma" and claims that the trauma parallels that of sexual abuse.[13] We all have times in our lives when we are shamed due to sexual expression or anatomy, but when a person expresses sexual orientation differences, a shame is experienced that exceeds what is felt by someone who is heterosexual. To explain this phenomenon, Kort coined the term "covert cultural sexual abuse." He defines covert cultural sexual abuse as "chronic verbal, emotional, psychological, and sometimes sexual assaults against an individual's gender expression, sexual feelings and behaviors."[14] Kort defines this behavior as "covert" because there are indirect and subtle messages, such as verbal and nonverbal assaults by others. To clarify, as Kort does in his book, he is not saying that those of different orientations have been sexually abused; he is saying that we need to understand the negative messages that society has inflicted, which are similar to abuse and harassment. Our culture tends to inundate us with messages from faith communities, political leaders, families, and schools that being gay or transgender is wrong and sinful. Children take these messages in, identify with them, and then carry shame and sexual wounding into their adult lives.

Omar came to therapy to discuss the struggle he'd been having due to his family's shock and disgust when he came out to them as a gay man. He had remained silent about being gay for a very long time. Omar was forty-four years old when he finally settled into his gay identity and began living with his partner. Omar's family was deeply religious, with strong traditions that included the extended family. Omar found, when gradually telling his family members, that some of his younger siblings and cousins were more open and accepting of his identity. However, Omar's parents expressed a great deal of shame and shock about their son's identity.

Coming to terms with the family's reaction took time for Omar. Therapy included work on anger and depression, as Omar had been hiding his true self for many years. In fact, Omar had not used safe sex practices during some of his early years due to the shame he felt and a denial of his own identity. He learned that his own self-hatred and internalized homophobia had led him down a dangerous path, as he didn't take care of himself sexually during his twenties.

The DVD *Fish Can't Fly* (see the resources section) was helpful for Omar, and eventually he shared it with his parents. Doing this led the family to a greater understanding of Omar's struggle with identity and acceptance from his family and God.

YOU'RE GOING TO GO BLIND!!

For most people, masturbation has a deep-rooted history of shame. We usually begin masturbating at a young age and a caregiver may have shamed us into keeping it a "dirty" secret. Although masturbation is normal and quite novel when we are children and start discovering our bodies, as we grow up, that shame remains. Masturbation is secret, hush-hush, and many people have difficulty even saying the word. When we get into a relationship, we usually don't discuss masturbation and may be embarrassed or ashamed if found masturbating.

Although masturbation gets such a bad rap in society, the reality is that it's actually very good for us! Under normal circumstances, masturbation is how we learn about our sexuality and it may have produced our first orgasm. When masturbation is not compulsive or excessive (interrupting one's level of functioning), it can have stress-relieving attributes, as well as health benefits. For women, orgasm increases blood flow to the vaginal area and helps keep the vulva and vagina healthy. When women masturbate on a regular basis, vaginal tissues are more moist and supple. Masturbation allows us to play with fantasy in a way that is healthy and appropriate. Some people believe that masturbation takes away from sex for a couple in a relationship, but it can actually enhance the sexual relationship. For men and women who have difficulty achieving orgasm, masturbation can be a way of learning about one's body and learning how to orgasm, if that is the person's goal. A couple who each find that masturbation is enjoyable will likely find that their desire responds to this increased focus on self-stimulation. Desire creates desire! Chapter 4 has more information about masturbation.

Lila and Logan came to their therapist with an issue regarding Logan's masturbation. Lila explained, "I discovered that Logan masturbates and this shocked me! I thought that, when we moved in together and were having sex on a regular basis—which we agree we are—that Logan wouldn't be masturbating anymore. I feel like I'm not satisfying him or something!" Logan responded by saying that he masturbates about three or four times a week and didn't know that this would be such an issue for Lila.

The therapist normalized this situation: masturbation is common, even when couples are married or living together. They discussed the advantages of masturbation, and Lila spoke of her own occasional self-stimulation. Thinking about the benefits of masturbation helped Lila feel more accepting of Logan's self-stimulation and allowed her to find the time for her own masturbation on a more regular basis.

HEALING SHAMEFUL SEXUAL WOUNDS

Healing from sexual wounds takes some work and a long, hard look at your own values and beliefs. This means putting aside the voices that have been telling you what is sexually right or wrong, as well as any coercion or violation that may have colored your own beliefs. Consider what your ideas are about sex and challenge the ones that compel you to be something you're not. Talk about what you need, what you want, and how you feel when it comes to sex. Don't settle for anything less than what you really want!

MOVING ACROSS THE BRIDGE

Not many people escape dealing with a sexual wound. Sexual wounds are part of the way we perceive our sexual selves, which is vital to the communication with our partners regarding sexuality, desires, needs, fears, and wants. Secrets are binding and stifling, so consciously looking at the secrets and working through them can play a big part in communicating about our sexual selves. Moving past this part of the bridge can be freeing and essential for sexual health.

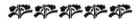

SEXERCISES

I. Grounding: when sexual abuse is occurring, some people will dissociate. Again, this is the tendency to "check out" in order to survive the abuse. Some survivors continue to dissociate when certain triggers occur in their lives. One trigger may be sex. If this is a problem for you or your partner, here are some ways to facilitate grounding, to allow you to be present in the moment, even during daily activities.

During daily activity:

- Touch an object, such as a rock, a piece of cloth, or something that is comforting to you, to experience some sensual feedback.
- Allow yourself to do a physical activity, such as stomping, clapping, readjusting your body, or exercising.
- Say a memorized poem or sing a familiar song.
- Describe in detail where you are and what you are doing.
- Call a friend. Talk about a funny story.
- Drink something cold or splash water on your face.
- Watch a funny movie.

During sexual activity:

- You may need a "safe" word or gesture to indicate that you need to stop the sexual activity.
- If you feel yourself having a flashback, stop your activity and pay attention to objects in the room. Talk to your partner about the need

to do this. Name objects, sounds, smells, and sensations so that you are grounded in the moment.

- Open your eyes and say your partner's name aloud. Repeat his or her name.
- After interrupting your sexual activity, you may not be able to return to an intense physical interaction. That's okay. You can then use some of the techniques under "during daily activity" to help yourself be in the moment.

II. Mindfulness (dealing with negative emotions and thoughts):

- When you have a negative thought, imagine a revolving door and allow that negative thought to go through the door; say "exit" as it passes on through.
- Another way to handle negative thoughts or self-talk is to imagine the thought as a message written in the sand and allow the waves to wash them away. Similarly, thoughts written on leaves can be blown away by the wind.
- Think about the negative messages that come to mind during sexual activity that are shame-based. Think about where the shame comes from. In your journal, write down the messages and think of positive or comforting messages to replace them. For example, "I wish he or she would hurry up and get off of me." Change this to "I am in a safe place and in control. I can get aroused and enjoy myself."

Note: *If you are feeling unsafe with your partner, this is not a good exercise for you. Try to establish ground rules that are explained in chapter 6. If this isn't helpful, see a therapist to work on the problem.*

III. Progressive muscle relaxation: anxiety tends to flood in when we are struggling with sexual wounds. Practice this sexercise often, until you can relax without the cues.

Find a quiet place with no distractions, removing contact lenses, if needed. This exercise can be done sitting in a comfortable chair or lying down. The key is to be as comfortable as possible. You can either use this text to do the exercise or use a recorder to record the text beforehand, then listen to it and follow the instructions.

Begin by allowing your eyes to close and taking a deep breath, breathing in through your nose and out through your mouth. Take two more deep breaths in this manner, thinking of calm and relaxation as you breathe in, then thinking of releasing tension and anxiety as you breathe out. Now, breathe normally . . .

We are going to tense and release muscles throughout the body, feeling the difference between tension and relaxation. When you tense different muscles, hold the tension in the muscle for about ten seconds. (When recording this script, allow time during the tensing of the muscles before reading on.) If tensing causes pain in any location, skip that muscle and move on to the next.

Let's begin at the forehead. Wrinkle up your forehead, as if you are raising your eyebrows. Hold that tension, paying attention to the sensation of your muscles being tight and tense. Allow your forehead to relax, paying close attention to the difference between the muscles feeling tense and the muscles feeling relaxed.

With your forehead muscle feeling relaxed, move to your eyes now. Close your eyes tightly, again noticing the tension. Release the tension, feeling the difference between being tense and being relaxed.

Move down to the mouth, opening your mouth wide, feeling the tension in those muscles around your mouth. Now relax those muscles, paying attention to the difference between tension and relaxation. Next, clamp your teeth shut, tight, to feel the tension in your jaw where you keep a lot of stress. Relax your jaw, feeling how different it feels from when it was tense.

Move to the neck area, moving your head back, noticing the tension. Let your neck return to its normal position. At this time, scan the muscles you have already tightened and relaxed. Allow yourself to notice any muscle that is tense. Release that muscle.

Now move to your shoulders. Shrug your left shoulder up toward your left ear, feeling the tension in your upper back, another place that we naturally hold in stress. Let that muscle relax, noticing the difference between being tense and relaxed. Do the same with the right shoulder.

Make a muscle with your left arm, like when you were a child and wanted to show someone your muscle. Release, then follow with your right arm.

Make a fist with your left hand, feeling the tension, then release and follow with your right hand.

Move to your torso, focusing on your chest. Take in a deep breath, holding that breath until it becomes uncomfortable, then release your breath slowly, feeling the relaxation. Often we hold our breath when we are tense. Feel how relaxing it is to let that breath release and become normal breathing.

Now, pay attention to your belly. Pull your belly in, as though you are trying to make your stomach look flat. Then release the tension, feeling the difference.

Move to the buttocks, tightening up your bottom. Feel that tension, then relax, feeling the difference between relaxation and tension.

Move to the lower legs and point your toes, feeling the tension. Then allow your toes to return to their normal position.

Next, flex your toes up toward your knees, feeling the tension through your calves. Release, noticing the difference between relaxation and tension.

Again, scan your body, re-tensing and releasing until your body feels more relaxed. Remain relaxed for a few minutes, then allow yourself to take in a deep breath.

When you exhale this time, allow yourself to relax even more, feeling your body sink down further into the chair or the bed. Let yourself feel relaxed for a period of time. When you are ready to get on with your day, count from five to one, allowing yourself to become more alert and aware of your surroundings as you count up to one.

IV. Sensate focus is explained in more detail in appendix C. This is a technique used in sex therapy for a number of sexual issues. This a good exercise to do when you are trying to establish a sexual relationship after trauma or after a difficult time working through trauma. As a couple, you can engage in sensate focus exercises at your own pace and with varying levels of intimacy. Stay at each level until both you and your partner feel comfortable moving to the next level. If you are struggling with anxiety, try the relaxation exercise in sexercise 3 (above) to reduce your anxiety before trying sensate focus.

If the thought of intimate touching causes you fear or discomfort, we want to suggest an excellent DVD, *Relearning Touch* by Wendy Maltz. This DVD establishes a safe, fun way of touching that builds from simple, almost child-like touch to more intimacy. See the resources section of this book for more information on this DVD.

Level I of Sensate Focus: Begin with clothes on or off and caress each other, front to back, head to toe. At this point, avoid the breasts and genitals. Both partners take turns giving and receiving caresses. Taking turns is necessary so each partner can concentrate fully on the sensations and the reaction of the other. If this kind of touch provokes anxiety or discomfort, simply begin at a point where you are comfortable. That may be holding hands, giving each other backrubs, or caressing each other's face. During this level, the focus is on the giver touching in a way he or she enjoys, avoiding anything that is uncomfortable to the receiver. The purpose of touch at this level is not to be sexual. Intercourse isn't a goal at this level. Talk with each other about your experience and what you found, both physically and emotionally.

Level II of Sensate Focus: This level incorporates Level I, but the focus includes the kind of touch the receiver wants. He or she shows the partner the touch that is enjoyable by guiding the hand and/or talking to the partner about what is enjoyable. Continue taking turns, prohibiting intercourse.

Level III of Sensate Focus: At this level, you and your partner continue the touching from the previous levels and now include the breasts and genitals. Continue to focus on the sensations and on communicating what is enjoyable and what each partner wants, and not on the goal of orgasm. The person being touched puts his or her hand on the other's hand, helping to apply pressure or a different pace. The person being touched is not to take over, but just add input about sensations and pleasure. Intercourse is not pursued.

Level IV of Sensate Focus: At this point, you are combining all the previous levels, enjoying the mutual touching and stimulation to the point of orgasm, if desired. The goal, at this level, can be intercourse if both partners are comfortable with this.

V. If you are struggling with your sexual orientation or have come out, but still find that there's shame involved, please take time to read about this. We have included some useful books in the resources section, and we encourage you to read and then discuss what you're feeling with your partner, friend, parents, or therapist. Also look for a support group in your area.

VI. Consider your attitudes about masturbation, thinking about where your attitudes came from in your past. Remember the many advantages to this very normal expression of sexuality. If you are comfortable discussing masturbation with your partner, you may want to talk about your habits and about the advantages of masturbation in your relationship.

4

EXPRESSIONS OF SEXUAL RESPONSE

Acknowledging Your Differences

My partner is always pushing me to initiate sex. What about the days
when we naturally just wanted the same thing?

—Female, age 52

- Do you and your partner have dissimilar sexual needs and express
  your sexual needs differently?
- Do you argue about what's "normal" and what's "necessary" in a
  sexual relationship?
- Is it difficult for you and your partner to compromise about sexual
  and relationship needs?
- Does it seem that, in the past, you and your partner agreed about
  desire and sexual frequency but now it feels like you're always either arguing about it or avoiding one another?

THE UNIQUE PATTERN OF OUR NEEDS

Every day in our therapy offices, we hear couples attempting to negotiate their differences. The stories of their lives are like different threads
in a tapestry. The threads are of various hues, thicknesses, and textures.

All tapestries are distinct, but when we examine them closely, we see that there are some common patterns. Most couples eventually find themselves tangled in the threads of each partner's uniqueness. They ask, "Why aren't you more like me?" "How could you possibly see things so differently from me?" "Why can't you change so that we are more alike?"

This dialogue about differences can lead couples down a treacherous path, filled with accusations and hurt. Power struggles about whose thoughts and feelings are "right" lead to barriers that block understanding. Each person's individuality is usually seen as exciting and intriguing during the beginning stages of a romantic relationship, and this uniqueness can be powerful. However, as the relationship continues year after year, the differences, which were initially so captivating, can become an irritant or aggravation.

The challenge in long-term relationships becomes learning to appreciate differences and not letting them stand in the way of intimacy and passion. In other words, the task becomes one of seeing that the dissimilar threads make up a more beautiful tapestry than if the threads were all exactly the same.

Let's look at some of the most common intimacy struggles for couples: sexual response differences, desire discrepancy, variations in arousal styles, the meaning of touch, and the balance of interdependence. Keep in mind that differences are not always along gender lines. Some males may have lower sexual desire than females, and some females may discover that their arousal pattern is more traditionally "masculine" than it is traditionally "feminine." Same-sex couples find that their shared gender doesn't necessarily protect them from the intimacy struggles of their straight peers, because we are individually unique.

SEXUAL HEALING

We're a gay couple and sometimes our straight friends will joke that we must have it easy since we're both men and, therefore, have a lot in common. We tell our friends that nothing could be further from the truth. We have some of the same problems that our straight friends complain about, like feeling disconnected at times, feeling like we don't communicate very well about our feelings. But we also have some unique issues since we *are* gay . . . like coming out as a couple to our parents, whether to show our affection openly, and whether to keep our relationship a secret to some people who aren't accepting of us. But my partner and I do enjoy the fact that, both being males, we seem to understand each other sexually pretty well.

There's a lot of wisdom in this observation! It's been found that we can't assume that "a couple is a couple," no matter the gender. Gay, lesbian, bisexual, and transgender (GLBT) couples have some similarities to straight couples, but they also have a uniqueness of their own. We find that no one is immune to the struggles of connecting and communicating. We all bring something unique to a relationship. Finding that you have differences in personality, needs, and desires (even though you are the same gender) necessitates open dialogue and learning to appreciate the uniqueness that you each bring to the relationship. We list some helpful books, DVDs, and websites in the resources section.

SEXUAL RESPONSE DIFFERENCES

In the 1950s and 1960s, William Masters and Virginia Johnson began researching the physiology of sexual response.[1] Before this time, no one had studied human sexual behavior in the laboratory setting. The team of Masters and Johnson studied heart rate over the sexual cycle, muscular contractions in the body during sexual response, and many other physiological reactions while study participants were engaged in sexual behavior.

Masters and Johnson described four stages of sexual response, which they termed *excitement, plateau, orgasm,* and *resolution.* We will describe these phases briefly, but keep in mind that there are many more subtle physiological reactions taking place. Additionally, the physical changes in each phase will differ for a variety of reasons, such as aging, illness, and medication usage.

The primary physiological process that occurs during the *excitement* phase is an increase of blood flow, or vasocongestion, to the genital area. In males, the dilation of the blood vessels produces an erection. In females, vasocongestion usually leads to lubrication of the vagina, engorgement of the clitoris, and swelling of the labia.

During the *plateau* phase of the sexual response cycle, vasocongestion reaches its peak. In males, the penis is completely erect and the testes draw up close to the body. In females, the most notable change during the plateau phase is the formation of the orgasmic platform, or the tightening of the outer third of the vagina. In both males and females, there is a further increase in the rate of breathing, blood pressure, and pulse. Muscles throughout the body begin to contract, heart rate and respiration quicken, and the nipples become erect.

For the male, *orgasm* consists of a series of rhythmic contractions of the pelvic organs, forcing the seminal fluid through the urethra. For females, orgasm is a series of rhythmic muscular contractions of the orgasmic platform and uterus. Females may have several small contractions in a mild orgasm, as many as a dozen in a very intense, prolonged orgasm, or more than one orgasm. In both males and females, there are sharp increases in blood pressure, pulse, and breathing rate during orgasm. Additionally, muscles contract throughout the body.

Following orgasm is the *resolution* phase, during which the body returns to its unaroused physical state. Resolution represents a reversal of the processes that build up during the first two phases. For females, this phase will take about fifteen to thirty minutes. There is a gradual return of blood pressure, pulse, and breathing rate to the unaroused levels. In males, loss of erection occurs following orgasm as they enter what is called the refractory period. During this period, males are incapable of being aroused again, having an erection, or experiencing an orgasm. The length of the refractory period varies considerably from one man to another and lasts longer as a man ages. Women don't enter a refractory period and some women are able to experience multiple orgasms.

As we can see, Masters and Johnson's four-stage model focused almost entirely on the physiological aspects of sexual response. Masters and Johnson didn't consider the constructs of desire and passion in their study. The omission of subjective feeling states is challenging because so often there are discrepancies between a person's physiological state and emotional state. For instance, a person can feel intense sexual desire, yet have no vaginal lubrication or erection. And, surprisingly, there may be indications of arousal, such as an erection, with insufficient levels of subjective desire.

Critics have pointed out that the Masters and Johnson model is problematic due to the selection process of female participants, resulting in a self-fulfilling outcome. To participate in the study, female subjects were required to have a history of orgasm through both intercourse and self-stimulation, thus having a high and consistent level of sexual desire. However, the general population of females in the United States does not report *consistently* high desire or ease of orgasm.[2] Additionally, the subjects in this study had to be comfortable with observation by laboratory staff and having physiological instruments attached to them, while engaging in sexual behavior! Therefore, it's unwise to assume that this model represents the response cycle of most females.

Helen Singer Kaplan expanded on the four-stage model, modifying it to include the component of desire, preceding arousal, orgasm, and resolution.[3] Physicians and therapists have used a linear model (desire, arousal, orgasm, and resolution) for years as the foundation for diagnosing and treating sexual dysfunctions and disorders for males and females.

It's not uncommon to hear a woman say, "I don't know what's wrong with me, but I would be perfectly happy to never have sex again!" After more consideration, the woman usually explains that she can remember, at one time, feeling attracted to her partner, looking forward to his or her sexual attention, and being easily aroused. When the sexual fire has gone out, women often feel a sense of guilt, loss, and possibly irritation, while their partner often feels rejected, confused, and angry. What's happened to her desire? Recently, physicians and therapists have realized that the linear model, which begins with desire, doesn't fit most women.

How did females stray so far away from the linear model of desire, arousal, orgasm, and resolution? What happened to that first stage of passion and desire? Recall that the female subjects for the Masters and Johnson research were studied in a lab and had high levels of desire and arousal, which is not typical of women. Fortunately, Dr. Rosemary Basson, a clinical professor in the Department of Psychiatry and the Department of Obstetrics and Gynecology at the University of British Columbia, has reconceptualized the sexual response cycle for women.[4]

Dr. Basson's model (see figure 1) explains that a woman will often go through her day in a *neutral sexual state*, in which she does not feel much desire or need for sex. According to this model, the woman then considers her own motivation to have sex, termed the *spin-offs*, such as the longing to feel loved or accepted. She may feel the commitment of her relationship or the desire to feel emotionally close as motivators to have sex. These personal motivators lead to the deliberate choice to *seek sexual stimulation*. Or

A Woman's Sex Response Cycle

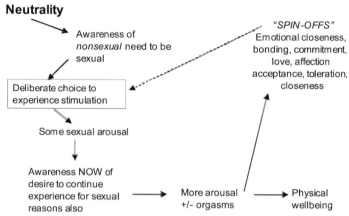

Figure 1.   A Woman's Sex Response Cycle.

Rosemary Basson, "The Female Sexual Response: A Different Model,"
Journal of Sex and Marital Therapy 26, no. 1 (2000): 51–65. Reprinted by
permission of the publisher (Taylor & Francis Group).

perhaps not. If a woman chooses to pursue sexual stimulation, it can lead
to *sexual arousal*. For example, she may receive clitoral stimulation, orally
or manually, and become aware of sexual arousal, such as lubrication or a
feeling of pressure and fullness in her pelvis. Arousal ushers in an awareness NOW of the *desire* to continue this stimulation for sexual reasons.
Arousal and desire may or may not progress to *orgasm* for the woman.
Even without orgasm, she may still experience a full sense of *emotional
and physical satisfaction*. Rather than linear, this model is circular, because the woman's sexual response loops back to the emotional motivators
that will likely lead her to desire sexual interaction in the future.

   The source of desire in women may be quite different from that in
men and arises from not only the innate hormonal drive, but more likely
from feelings that are not explicitly sexual. A woman's reasons for sexual
interaction are many and don't necessarily include the desire for genital
tension relief. The expectation of sexual pleasure may not even be a
motivator. Instead, a woman will consider many emotional, physical,
relational, and psychological factors when she chooses to seek sex.

   When women see the Basson model of female sexual response, their
eyes light up! One young woman stated, "I'm putting this diagram on my
refrigerator for my boyfriend to see so that he'll hopefully understand
me better!" Women don't necessarily begin their sexual journey at the

exact same place as men. Desire is not always the first order of business. That's okay! With healthy communication, adequate sexual techniques, and a trusting, safe environment, arousal and desire can be a part of a woman's sexual relationship.

It's not advisable to generalize the Basson model of neutrality to *all* women and at *all* times. Some women do follow the linear path of desire, arousal, orgasm, and resolution. This is particularly true for women who are young or in new, exciting, fresh relationships. This fact can lead to confusion for couples. A woman who is in a long-term relationship may miss the feeling of passion and sexual anticipation that she felt at the onset of the relationship. We'll look at the neurochemical foundation for this fact in the next section, "Desire Discrepancy."

Males tend to follow the four-stage linear model and to be innately driven for sexual pleasure, due to higher and more consistent levels of testosterone than women have. However, men may also have sexual challenges in each of the four stages. These sexual difficulties will be discussed throughout the book, but are explained in more detail in appendix A.

Although males and females tend to have differences in sexual response, some people report that they don't need or want an orgasm with every sexual encounter in order to feel a sense of well-being and sexual satisfaction. It may be challenging to believe that orgasm is not the goal for every sexual interaction. However, a couple can feel a sense of relief to discover that sensual connection may be more important and meaningful than striving for orgasm. Without performance pressure, couples can find comfort in erotic intimacy, with or without orgasm.

SEXUAL HEALING

My partner and I are definitely not in the same place when it comes to sexual desire! He seems to be in the mood for sex much more often than I am. I also find that it's so easy for him to orgasm and it's so much more complicated for me. Maybe if I could get there faster or more easily, I would also be in the mood more often. Just intercourse alone never leads to orgasm for me. What's going on?

This a good point! And it's fairly common that women find they don't orgasm by the thrusting movement of intercourse alone. Men are usually

*able to receive the right amount of stimulation and friction during inter-
course to achieve orgasm. For most females, however, stimulation of the
clitoris is necessary. Many intercourse positions don't provide adequate
rubbing of the clitoral area. Adding manual stimulation or a vibrator
along with intercourse will probably help.*

*We want to encourage you to examine how important your own orgasm
is for you. This can put a lot of pressure on a woman! Not all women
feel the need to orgasm and might feel very satisfied, both sexually and
emotionally, without orgasm. Chapter 9 goes into more depth regarding
various sexual positions and turn-ons for you and your partner.*

DESIRE DISCREPANCY

Couples often speak of their differences in sexual desire. It's more common that females report lower libido than do males; however, some
males also report suffering from low desire. For either gender, the lowered libido may be due to relational factors, such as miscommunication,
unresolved hostility, guilt, or specific turn-ons (i.e., a dependency on
porn, a fetish). Low sexual desire may also have a physical basis, such as
hormone changes, medication, illness, stress, fatigue, or aging issues.

Why Are We Different?

Males and females learn about their bodies in very different ways
when growing up. With male genitals being external and female genitals
being primarily internal, males discover their sexual arousal more easily than do females. Males are more likely to masturbate than females,
and males who masturbate do so more frequently than females who
masturbate. This is an important point because masturbation can play a
significant role in the development of sexual drive and response. In puberty, males learn that they can have an automatic and reliable erection,
which likely leads easily to orgasm. However, females may be unaware
of their subtle signs of sexual arousal and avenues to pleasure. Females
then have a dimmer awareness than males of their erotic signals from
their genitals.

Because most males masturbate, it's likely that they are "in touch" with their sexual stimulation needs. "On the other hand," females will find that masturbation can lead to increasing knowledge about their arousal. We recommend trying your hand at self-stimulation in order to enhance desire!

Masturbation . . . Sex with Someone You Love . . .

Masturbation can lead to an expansion of pleasurable behavior, enhanced orgasms, stress relief, and increased sexual desire. It can promote relaxation and sleep. Masturbation can boost mood with the release of endorphins. It's certainly safe sex!

For women only: In contrast to males, most females are not encouraged to masturbate, and masturbation isn't something most adolescent girls talk about with one another. But there's a lot that can be learned about one's body, G-spot, clitoris, sexual needs, and responses when you take matters into your "own hands." Find a comfortable and private place to explore.

- We encourage you, in chapter 2, to take a look at your genitals with a mirror. Explore them now with touch and identify the clitoris and inner and outer lips (labia).
- The clitoris has only one purpose, that of producing excitement and pleasure. The part of the clitoris that you can see is only the small, rounded, pea-sized knob of flesh just below the mons. If you push back the hood, or soft fold of skin covering, you can see the clitoral glans.
- The clitoris varies in size and is actually partially contained internally. Included as part of the clitoris are clitoral "legs," nine to eleven centimeters long, that spread back into the body and vestibular bulbs made up of erectile tissue.[5] Together these sensitive areas of the vulva become filled with blood during arousal. You may feel a sense of fullness or pressure in your pelvic area.
- Take your time as you touch your body . . . lower belly, breasts, inner thighs, pubic mons area.
- Stroke the vaginal lips and touch your clitoris. Lubricant can be added and you may find, with additional rubbing, that you produce your own lubrication. Stimulating the anterior wall of the vagina may lead you to the discovery of the G-spot area.

- Focus on any area that you find brings you more excitation and pleasure. Rub these areas repeatedly and rhythmically.
- Fantasize or read erotica.
- You might begin to feel some pelvic muscular tension, and you may want to flex those muscles.
- As the pleasure mounts, you may experience one or more orgasms. You might feel your muscles clenching, a pleasurable rush and release, and rhythmic contractions of the vaginal area and uterus.
- Don't worry about producing an orgasm. It may not happen easily and might take practice. This is an important step in learning about pleasure and arousal.
- Because self-stimulation increases sexual awareness, it can help you feel better about your body, genitals, and sexual response. You may want to share your experience with your partner to recreate the intensity and pleasure that you discovered on your own.

For men only: Grab on and go for it! No, really, here's the deal:

- Males masturbate by hand stimulation, rubbing on various objects, and humping.
- Most men use the technique of circling the hand around the shaft of the penis and using an up-and-down motion to stimulate the shaft and glans of the penis.
- Be sure to use some type of lubrication, such as soapsuds, lubricant, or saliva.
- Fantasy is helpful to increase arousal.
- Usually men increase the speed of stimulation as they approach orgasm.
- When a man comes, he often grips the shaft of the penis tightly.
- Immediately after orgasm, the glans and corona are very sensitive, and a man will usually avoid further stimulation.

Where Did Our Love Go?

Jan came to therapy by herself. Although Jan was past menopause, she was also a runner and in great physical shape. She talked about the sadness she felt in her relationship of ten years. Her partner, Jessica, didn't seem as interested in sex as she had once been. This caused Jan a lot of confusion and frustration because *she* still had a strong sex drive and fantasized about sex regularly. She found that staying in good physical condition also helped her to feel accepting of her body and to feel energized to have sex. She talked about the fact that Jessica was aware that her own libido had lessened in the past five years, and she felt she was letting Jan down. Jan missed the sexual intensity that she and Jessica both felt at the beginning of their relationship. She wondered what it might be like to look for someone else, someone more sexually compatible.

This is a common situation: differing sex drives between partners and finding that romantic love and passion wane with time. Sometimes we lament the loss of the stage in our relationship that was filled with passion and eroticism. Desire discrepancy then gets tangled up in feelings of resentment and hurt because we might interpret it as personal rejection. It's hard to accept that we have different sex drives. As therapists, this is probably the most common sexual complaint we hear. What do we suggest to these couples? Sometimes "no" is "no." Sometimes we just need to accept that the difference is there and try something like mutual masturbation. Or the person with low desire may just want to watch! Chapter 9 has some tips to help facilitate arousal.

VARIATIONS IN AROUSAL STYLES

Dana described that she felt more easily aroused if she could have her partner, Darrin, talk to her and look at her while making love. Dana liked active and invigorating interaction prior to and during sex. Darrin admitted that he found Dana's style to be distracting. He had discovered that he needed to concentrate on his own arousal and wanted to keep his eyes closed and be more internally focused during sex. This had become an increasingly important sexual interaction style for Darrin as he had begun to struggle with erectile issues. He found that his erection was more predictable if he focused on his own stimulation and physical needs.

Metz and McCarthy write about arousal patterns and point out the need to accept that healthy couples appreciate flexibility in arousal styles.[6] Three different styles are noted: partner interaction (focusing on the partner, active, eyes open, talkative, and energetic); self-entrancement (focusing on one's own body, eyes closed, quiet, routine and stylized touch); role enactment (role-play, fantasy, variety, experimentation).

How do we negotiate these different arousal styles? It may be frustrating or difficult to talk about, but it's important to make our needs known to each other. If our arousal styles are very different, we'll need to discuss having times that each can enjoy his or her own unique style and other times that we blend the styles enough to each find sensual satisfaction. These arousal styles are not fixed systems, but may change over time, with age, or with sexual needs. We need to be open to our partner's needs and our own.

 SEXUAL HEALING

I've been with my partner for twenty-five years and I have always wanted to try new types of sexual encounters. I'd like my partner to be willing to role-play something with me or to use a vibrator or to watch me stimulate myself. I think this would help my arousal since I've noticed that I need a bit more excitement as I age. I'm not sure my partner will go along with this and I don't even know how to ask her.

Your point is well taken. With age, it's not uncommon that people find that they need to add or change something about sexual stimulation in order to feel or maintain arousal. Don't be embarrassed about this fact, but be sensitive to your partner's own unique needs, both emotionally and sexually. It's usually better to have these types of conversations outside of the bedroom and not just before having sex. Give your partner time to think about your revelation and suggestions. It would be good to start by letting your partner know how much she means to you and what positive feelings you have about the sex that you've been having all these years. Then ask her to consider some of your desires with the stipulation that she can veto anything and everything. I know that doesn't sound like a compromise, but when it comes to sex, coercion has no place in the negotiation. You both can discuss what it would be like to explore some of your interests. You can also ask about hers. You may find that you intensely enjoy some erotic interaction or toy, but it's not necessary to engage in that activity every time. Be flexible about your requests and open-minded about hers. Having your partner read this book with you will be helpful, as she needs to know that she has her own voice.

❀❀ ❀❀ ❀❀

THE MEANING OF TOUCH

"He only touches me when he wants sex." "I'm afraid to touch her because she thinks that I will want to be sexual." "I'm not in the mood for sex all the time, but I'd love to just sit and cuddle or even kiss deeply." Do these statements sound familiar? We often have different feelings about or interpretations of touch in our relationships. Touch can become so filled with anxiety in a relationship that we avoid one another all together.

> Mandy and Mike came into therapy together to talk about the decline in their sexual frequency. They both agreed that they weren't having sex as often as before, and Mike felt that they were avoiding each other at all costs. Mandy confirmed that Mike's perception was accurate; she didn't want him to touch her because she felt pressure that his touch and her response would cause Mike to think that the touching would lead to sex at that moment. Mandy wanted to have more physical contact, even sensual contact, but didn't always want it to lead to sex. She explained, "Mike, I feel really uncomfortable when you come up behind me when I'm at the sink and you put your hands between my legs or start rubbing me!" Mike agreed that this had been a common way he approached Mandy, but replied that he had stopped all touching now that Mandy had become so distant.

It's difficult to stay connected emotionally and sexually when there's very little touch of any kind. It is especially challenging to move from almost no touching to intimate erotic touching. Touch is an important aspect of any relationship; it's calming and shows compassion, and it can also indicate desire and arousal. Touch is so important that some people have confessed that they go to a massage therapist just so they can feel that reassuring touch on their body, especially when they are not receiving this at home.

Take some time to talk to each other about what touch means in your intimate relationship. Incorporate all types of touch so that the connection stays strong. There are many kinds of touch that lovers have, and they don't all have to lead to sex. There's affectionate, soothing, calming, and loving touch. There's playful, interactive, non-erotic touch. Sensual and erotic touch can include genital touching or light massage of other areas of the body. Sensual caressing of various areas of the body can lead to arousal and erotic stirrings. Dancing, showering or bathing together, cuddling in bed, long and close hugging, or even making out can all be great ways to stay physically connected through touch without feeling that this interaction needs to lead to sex. However, we need to be able to talk openly about the meaning of touch so there is no misinterpretation regarding what the interaction is about.

 ## SEXUAL HEALING

My partner and I have been giving each other very mixed signals, I think. He says that I'm cold and never in the mood to have sex, unless I'm drinking. I think he may be right. I don't want him to think that I need to drink in order to have sex with him, but I am so uncomfortable with his touch. He tries to snuggle with me on the couch or he'll touch me between my legs when we're driving some place, and this sort of freaks me out. He says he's not trying to force or pressure me to have sex, but I feel like he wants more and so I back off. I don't want to lose him, but I'm not sure what to do.

You've brought up several really good points. First, sometimes people get in the habit of loosening up for sex by using alcohol. While a little alcohol may make you less inhibited, it can lead to a dependence on drinking to make you feel comfortable with sex. And then you're not really "present," are you?

Second, when your partner tells you that he's not trying to pressure you to have sex, that may very well be true. It's understandable that it would be hard to trust that your partner is touching just to stay connected, but it's important to talk to him about your distrustful feelings and allow him to understand your fears or hesitancy.

And this brings us to a third point. It might be that your partner does want to be sexual when he's touching you, but that he would forgo his desires, at that time, and just enjoy the intimacy of touching. For instance, your partner might say, with all honesty, that when he touches you between your legs, he's turned on, maybe fantasizing about more, but that he'll be okay if that's all it is.

Finally, it would be worthwhile to think about what sex means to you. Consider what you like about being sexual with your partner. Avoiding sex can lead to a great deal of awkwardness, so talk with your partner about what you'd like in terms of sex. But make it clear that you want touch for the sake of affection and closeness and that you'd like to clearly express when you want touch that leads to sex. Communicate openly because mixed messages about touch lead to hurt and sometimes anger.

THE BALANCE OF INTERDEPENDENCE

How much togetherness is healthy? How much time do we need to share with each other in order to have a strong relationship? Will too much closeness interfere with sexual tension and passion? The answers to these questions are complex. Couples are made up of individuals with their own unique needs for dependency and independency. Some couples come together so closely that they are rarely seen apart. And then other couples seem to live very separate lives, perhaps only seeing each other on rare occasions due to shift work or hectic schedules.

What's healthy, then, when it comes to closeness, and how does this relate to sex? It appears that we need a good dose of each other and intimacy while still having some separateness and independence. This is a tall order when it comes to long-term relationships! Too much intimacy and togetherness may feel smothering or engulfing to some of us, while others express they are lonely even in their long-term relationship.

Landon came to therapy with concern that he and his partner, Leslie, were rarely sexual. He related that the initial stages of their relationship were filled with passion and sexual energy. Landon remembered that he and Leslie would find time in the middle of their very busy lives to meet, almost anywhere and anytime, to have sex. Leslie and Landon also had great chemistry when it came to talking about their lives, everything from the mundane daily details of life to their dreams for the future. Landon explained that the emotional connection continued now, but both he and Leslie felt they had become such good friends that being sexual seemed oddly too familiar.

Leslie joined Landon for couples therapy and they both agreed that they loved the emotional intimacy and closeness that they shared, but missed the exciting unpredictable heat of their early passion. With the help of therapy, Landon and Leslie explored ways to turn the heat up. They would have preferred to leave sexual encounters up to spontaneity and chance, but they determined that they would have to plan for sexual dates. They had let their children and work interfere to the point that they were talking about these issues constantly, and they desperately needed time away to relax and enjoy each other again.

Leslie asked Landon if they could each take a week and plan something surprising and special for the other. He loved this idea and it led to some inventive ways to have fun and spice up their sexual encounters. This reminded them of the dating stage of their relationship because it required that they each spend time thinking of ways to surprise and enjoy each other.

Each of us needs to examine what emotional closeness does or doesn't do for the sexual relationship. Sexual desire may be enhanced by emotional connection, or the psychological intimacy that bonds us may actually interfere with passion and eroticism. If emotional closeness hampers the expression of the erotic, we need to explore ways to enhance playfulness and mystery in order to generate some heat. This requires us to explore surprise and unpredictability; steering away from the routine and the expected can bring spice and heat to the table.

SEXUAL HEALING

My partner and I have been together for several years and we don't seem to have much in common any more. We don't talk much. We don't argue. We don't spend time together. We hardly ever go out together now. In fact, we usually just come home from work and do our own thing. She likes to watch certain TV shows and I get on the computer, check my financial situation, and read newspapers online. We respect each other. I think she's brilliant; she's a physician. And she seems to admire my knowledge about the stock market. But we're not having much sex now either. We're just living two very separate lives. What should we do?

It's great that you can identify the strengths in your relationship! You admire and respect one another. You don't have conflict. Sit down soon with your partner—no TV, no computer, just the two of you. You might bring up the conversation with something like, "I feel like we've become so distant and I miss you. It seems we've gotten into a rut with work and commitments. I'd love to spend time with you! Can we talk about some of the things that we used to do when we were first together?" There must have been activities that you both enjoyed when dating. If you two can come up with some things from the past or even take on some new hobbies or activities together, you'll find the shared time may bring back some of the sexual interest that you once had. Think about shared fun activities: cooking, dancing close, hiking near a quaint bed-and-breakfast, or even redecorating the bedroom.

Keep in mind that you both need to talk about how to find each other again . . . both outside the bedroom and in the bedroom. Sharing your lives will help, but you'll also need to make sex a priority again. Plan some relaxing time that will allow you two to enjoy shared activities, but also will give you the ability to focus on each other sexually.

MOVING ACROSS THE BRIDGE

It's challenging to realize that you and your partner have so many potential differences. However, it's inevitable that your uniqueness will appear and it's better to be prepared and to know something about yourself as you cross this area of the bridge. Whether it is sexual response differences, desire discrepancies, variations in arousal styles, differences in the meaning of touch, or an imbalance in interdependence, you and your partner can communicate about these issues and find solutions to the challenges.

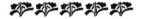

SEXERCISES

I. Think about the linear sexual response model (desire, arousal, orgasm, and resolution). Do you find that you or your partner fits this model as it relates to arousal? Alternatively, do you or your partner fit the Basson neutrality model?

To help you determine if and when you may feel some desire or yearning for sex, try the following from Barbach's book[7]:

For the next three days, make several notes in your journal regarding your level of desire during the day. A high level of desire would be ranked at a 10; a low level of desire would be ranked at a 0 or 1. Beside the ranking, write down the time of day. Additionally, note what you were doing or thinking at the time you "took your reading." Example:

7:30 a.m. "1" Got out of the shower and inspected my weight gain!

10:00 a.m. "5" Received a compliment from my coworker about my hair and outfit.

6:00 p.m. "7" Went for a run after work and felt stronger and more positive about my legs and weight control.

7:00 p.m. "2" Stressed out with the kids, supper dishes, messy house.

9:30 p.m. "7" Partner helped with the house, supported my exercise program, rubbed my back after the shower.

Examine your notes alone and share them with your partner, if you feel comfortable doing this. The following are the values of this exercise:

• You can look at the specific time of day when you might feel some desire and arousal—this might be a time to pursue sex or a sensual massage with your partner.
• You can examine your thoughts and behaviors at the times of desire and arousal and ask yourself, "What turns me on?"
• You can see that desire fluctuates—you may feel more desire or arousal at certain times. It's not always a constant.
• You can learn that you are not always a "1" or "10" and your partner isn't always the opposite. You may have thought that he or she was always a "10," but you discover that his or her desire fluctuates, as does yours.

II. Males and females learn about their bodies and sexual responses in very different ways. If you are a female, you may not have ever really had a chance to see what your vulva looks like. Give yourself permission to explore your genital area, using a mirror. This will allow you to become familiar with the structures of your genitals. Take the time to investigate your anatomy and the sources of pleasure and sensuality.

There are resources in the back of this book that will aid you in identifying different anatomical structures. Talk to your physician if you find that you have any pain or discomfort.

III. Recall the three styles of sexual arousal: partner interaction; self-entrancement; role-enactment. Think about which arousal style describes you best right now.

Partner Interaction: talking with your partner, having your eyes open, and being aware of your partner's reactions.

Self-Entrancement: keeping your eyes closed, having a keen awareness of your own physical sensations, being quiet, and concentrating.

Role-Enactment: experimenting, role-playing, using toys, and sharing fantasies.

Talk with your partner about these three styles and examine how you both feel about them. Do you accept each other's style? Do you feel that another style would suite you better individually or as a couple? Would you like to try something different?

IV. Touch is a critically important aspect of an intimate relationship. Think about how you and your partner used to touch and how you touch now. Think about all the different types of touch: affectionate, playful, sensual, and passionate. Talk to each other about what types of touch you are missing in your relationship. Talk about ways to incorporate more touch in your relationship and if your schedule permits it. If there is little time for touching, talk about what you can do to make room for each other.

V. Some couples prefer more space between them and other couples like to spend a lot of time together. Think about what you would like when it comes to time alone and time with your partner. Keep a log of each day of the week, broken down into hours. Look at the time you are spending in different endeavors. How much time do you spend with your partner? Ask your partner to do the same. Discuss what you each want. Do you want and need more time together? Is there a way to bring more togetherness into your schedule? Do you need more time alone or more privacy?

5

ACCEPTANCE OF LIFE'S CHALLENGES

Affirming Your Journey

I feel like our sex life has changed in a negative way since my diabetes diagnosis. I feel responsible because sex is much more complicated now and we're growing distant.

—Male, age 44

- Do moods affect your sexual relationship?
- What effects do sexual disorders have on your relationship?
- How does childbirth and being a parent affect you as a sexual person?
- Are you having side effects from illness, cancer, or medications that affect your sexual desire or arousal?
- Do you understand the influence that age is having on your body, your emotions, and your sexual relationship?

Menopause, aging, illness, sexual dysfunction, psychological problems, childbirth, and medications can all be "mood killers" in the bedroom. The image of romantic, wild, passionate sex goes out the window, and in the door come dry vaginas, flaccid penises, low desire, and all kinds of other "real life" mood killers that get into bed with a couple. The good news is that although body changes are inevitable, they don't mean death to one's sex life. The important elements of adjusting successfully to life's changes are keeping a dialogue going, affirming each other's needs, remembering to be creative, and understanding limitations.

> Nick, a thirty-one-year-old man, was put on antidepressants by his health-care provider after a particularly difficult bout with depression. Nick also sought therapy to help overcome his depression, at his doctor's request. He told his therapist that his partner was upset about their relationship, but wouldn't be more specific. When the therapist asked how things were going for the couple sexually, Nick's head dropped. He quietly said that he was having difficulty in that area. After some gentle questioning, the therapist realized that Nick was having erection problems, which are a common side effect of the antidepressant. The therapist referred Nick back to his health-care provider, and he was given an antidepressant that did not have this side effect. Nick's erectile problem dissipated, and he was able to work on his depression as well.

CHILDBEARING YEARS

Couples often complain of being too tired to have sex because of over-whelming schedules, homework to oversee, and baths to organize before bedtime. Pregnancy, childbirth, infertility, and raising children can all be stressors on a sexual relationship.

In pregnancy, physical and hormonal changes take place. This might be hard to understand for the partner and the pregnant woman. These changes can cause avoidance of sex for both partners and can lead to nine months of resentment about sex and lack of attention if both are not communicating feelings to each other. By opening the lines of communication, partners can make pregnancy a bonding experience, instead of a distancing event. Remember, sex is possible and important for a relationship throughout pregnancy, but it's necessary to be creative with positions and techniques during different trimesters.

How about after the baby is born? Most women feel far from sexy due to extra weight, lack of sleep, breastfeeding, and being buried deep in poopy diapers. The sexual relationship is going to change, no matter how we look at it. Be supportive of each other, and most importantly, talk, talk, TALK! This can be a very rewarding and positive time of life. Be sure to make time for each other.

Bob and Belinda spoke in therapy about conflict they were having in the bedroom. Belinda described feeling sexually rejected by Bob and wondered if her C-section scar and saggy boobs were a turn-off for Bob. She talked about how she had become tired of initiating sex and being turned down night after night. Bob claimed that their hectic schedules with four kids' sports, band events, and late-night homework assignments kept him exhausted. Belinda became angry and questioned Bob about his time away from their family with his biking buddies. This led to Bob becoming defensive and mentioning that Belinda was no longer taking care of herself or the home. Through therapy, which included learning to communicate more effectively, they found that it was important to carve out time to be sexual and playful with each other. Bob and Belinda decided to take turns planning sexual dates and initiating sex.

SEXUAL HEALING

My partner seems to be more interested in our children than she is in me! I have complained, but she becomes defensive and says I'm selfish. I feel like I need her and that she doesn't really need me. Our sexual relationship is suffering. What can I do?

You are describing a common problem for couples. This is a touchy subject because mothers often feel an intense bond with and need to take care of their children. However, this bond needs to be balanced with a strong relationship with their partners. Try saying something like this: "I really feel left out of the mix. I'm scared that your time with the kids is pulling us apart. What can I do to help you? I really miss our time together." Talking about your feelings and offering to help sets the stage for further explorations of important emotions for both of you. Be sure to get a sitter now and then and spend alone time without the kids. Talk about your future, your dreams, and your desires; not kids, bills, and home repairs.

An intimate relationship should not fall to the bottom of a person's "to do list" when they have children. Sex is an important aspect of a relationship, but not always one of the priorities for couples with a family. Time alone should occur on a regular basis. We often hear couples complain that they can't get a sitter. Looking at it in a more creative way, the kids can be put to bed, a picnic can be enjoyed on the bedroom floor, and time together can happen anyway. Sex may have to be scheduled; if not, it won't happen. Once the couple gets in the mood, there will be no concern about whether it had to be planned!

Having kids can be a strain on one's sex life, but not having kids when a couple wants them can be a problem, too. Infertility problems can be difficult and devastating. According to research, about one in seven women experiences problems with fertility, but approximately half of that number will eventually succeed in conceiving.[1] Most infertility problems can be linked to a medically defined cause; however, no cause can be found in about 3 percent of the cases.

What can a couple do when sex becomes a means to an end with a disappointing outcome? The couple might try taking a few months off from having sex only to have a baby, and shift to having sex to enjoy each other and reconnect. It's important not to listen to the opinions of busybodies, who all have stories about their sister's or their hairdresser's infertility problems. Couples with infertility issues are often plagued with offensive questions about when they are going to have children, which compound the feelings of inadequacy and sadness. The couple needs to remain conscious of how to connect emotionally and sensually in order to remain intimate partners.

 SEXUAL HEALING

I'm unable to conceive a child due to failure to ovulate. I just don't feel like having sex, and my partner doesn't understand. I don't even understand. Can you help?

This is a very frustrating problem. Sex becomes the means to having a baby, instead of an act of connection for two people. There is a lot of pressure to reproduce for you, your partner, and even family members and society. It's not uncommon for one or both partners to begin avoiding sex. Sexual contact becomes a painful reminder of what you are longing for, instead of being pleasurable. You may begin to define yourself through your inability to conceive a baby. It's really hard to focus on sexy thoughts when you are feeling all these emotions. If there are medical procedures being utilized to help with fertility, ask your health-care provider if the treatment may be interfering with your sexual desire. Talk to your partner; the intimacy of ongoing conversations can bring you together instead of distancing you.

WHEN ILLNESS STRIKES . . .

When illness strikes and a diagnosis is given, we are probably not thinking about how the illness is going to affect our sex life. However, sexual difficulties may plague men and women who suffer from various illnesses, such as diabetes, heart disease, cancer, hormone imbalance, high blood pressure, neurological disease, mental disorders, and gynecological and urological issues. As time goes on and there is acceptance of the diagnosis, couples often begin to come to terms with how the illness and the treatments are affecting their sexuality.

Not only can illness affect sexuality, but problems with sexuality can indicate underlying health issues. Low desire for women may be a sign of thyroid or other hormonal troubles. Painful sex can be a symptom of pelvic concerns. For men, erectile dysfunction can be a warning of possible physical disease. We need to be wise about our body and mindful about what our body is saying to us.

How many people really feel sexy when they are ill? As we've pointed out, illness can be a "mood killer," not to mention the side effects of medications and treatments. This can be a time of redefining the meaning of sex and how sex fits into one's life. Many factors come into play: body image, decreased energy, decreases in arousal and desire, and the effects of medication, as well as dealing with the emotional impact of how the illness is going to affect the rest of our lives. More than ever, there has to be dialogue with one's support group, partner, and healthcare provider. Often patients and doctors seem to have trouble discussing sex. It may be necessary for couples to shop around for a health-care provider who is sensitive to sexual problems. There is more about discussing sexual issues with one's doctor in chapter 11.

Of course, illness affects sex; but sex can also affect illness in a positive way. Sometimes the best medicine *is* sex! There are benefits to the cardiovascular workout that occurs during sex (it's important to check with a health-care provider to be sure it's safe). The touch and the muscular release during orgasm can be relaxing and help us sleep more deeply. We also benefit from the intimate closeness of our partner. Masturbation can bring some of the same health benefits, and it reminds us that we do have a degree of control over experiencing pleasure in our own bodies.

Tips for Redefining Sex during Illness

- Plan sex around the times you feel your best during the day. If you have difficulty after a long day, try to plan sex in the morning.
- If you need to take pain medication, take it about thirty minutes before having sex so pain is not an issue.
- Try different positions or techniques to make sex more comfortable.
- Talk to your partner about your feelings regarding your illness and sex; listen to your partner's feelings. More than likely, your partner is struggling, too.
- Touch outside of having sex. Hold hands, hug, touch each other gently.
- If there are times you physically cannot have sex, talk to your partner. Is mutual masturbation a possibility? Can you masturbate each other? Would sex toys help? You and your partner may have to be creative, or simply decide that sex is not an option at this time. It must be addressed either way.

Drug Effects

- Antihypertensives, used to regulate blood pressure, can decrease libido and cause problems achieving orgasm.
- Different hormones affect libido, either decreasing or increasing sexual desire.
- Drugs that are used for psychological problems can cause low libido and difficulty achieving orgasm.
- Opiates can decrease libido and cause difficulty achieving orgasm.

The best rule of thumb is this: when a new medication is prescribed and there are difficulties with sex, it's important to talk to a health-care provider. There may be a different drug you can use or a way to resolve the problem.

🌸 SEXUAL HEALING

I am in a lesbian relationship. My partner is depressed and suffering from an anxiety disorder. She never wants to have sex with me anymore. I'm sorry she feels bad, but this is ruining our relationship. I'm ready to give up.

We understand that you must be feeling very frustrated. Try to keep in mind that your partner is going through difficult times right now, but you also have to take care of your own emotional well-being. Anxiety and depression tend to be disorders in which a person seems to be self-focused. In other words, when a depressed or anxious person feels that bad, it's difficult to see outside his or her own pain and angst. A therapist might help, as well as a physical exam to be sure your partner doesn't have a health problem. Try couples therapy; look for someone who will be sensitive to a lesbian relationship. Talk to your partner about how she thinks you can be helpful in making her feel more comfortable about sex and express that you miss your sexual relationship with her. Avoid making her feel guilty, as guilt is a symptom of depression and counter-productive to getting a sexual relationship back on its feet. Most of all, don't take it personally; it's not you. Do something nice for yourself—go out with friends or take a class. Being around a depressed person can be draining, so getting away now and then will help you to re-energize. Try to exercise together, at least go for a walk. Chemically, exercise gets our endorphins going, which releases serotonin and helps us feel better. Besides that, the exercise will help your partner feel as though she has accomplished something, getting her out of the depressed "rut" that traps us when we suffer from depression.

A Broken Heart and Stroke

Heart disease and stroke can affect sexual activity in a number of ways, both emotionally and physically. When the severity of heart problems increases, sex may become dangerous due to the changes in heart rate and blood pressure. Problems such as breathing difficulty and chest pain can occur with intercourse, in conjunction with certain disorders of the heart.

Emotional concerns and fear of death become stumbling blocks for both partners when it comes to having sexual experiences after a stroke or heart disease has been diagnosed. Depression is a normal reaction for stroke and heart patients, which may put a damper on sex. The American Heart Association tells us that, although depression is common, in 85 percent of cases the average length of depression that is due to a reaction to heart disease is about three months.[2] A cardiologist should always be consulted regarding sexual encounters if heart disease is an issue. Keep in mind that for the most part, with the blessing of a physician, a satisfying sexual relationship can be realized after heart attack, stroke, or surgery.

As in other types of illness, the medication used to treat the disorder might affect sexuality. With all side effects from medication, keep an open dialogue with a health-care provider. There may be other drugs or treatments that can be used instead of the medication that is causing the side effects. Drugs such as Viagra, Cialis, and Levitra may be added to counter the effect of erectile dysfunction. It must be cautioned that these drugs mixed with nitrates have proven to be deadly cocktails; therefore, a physician should be consulted regarding how to use these drugs safely.

The American Heart Association assures heart patients that resuming an active sex life is possible. The following guidelines are recommended:

- Choose a familiar place that is free from distraction.
- Allow time after meals to ensure digestion.
- Pick a time that is more relaxed and when there is a feeling of being rested.
- Take medications before sex, if necessary.

Following a stroke, it's recommended that a person should be conscious of his or her feelings regarding any physical changes, such as paralysis, loss of sensation, weakness, and changes in body awareness. These physical changes may make previous sexual positions impossible to enjoy. New positions, toys, and perhaps pillows to support the affected areas of the body can optimize the sexual experience.

Heart disease and stroke bring new challenges to couples in the area of sexual intimacy. With a physician's guidance and continued communication between the couple, sensuality and physical connection can remain a vital part of the relationship.

Cancer

When a person is first diagnosed with cancer, sexual satisfaction and interaction may be the last thing on a couple's mind. For some people, sex is associated with health, vitality, and reproduction, while a cancer diagnosis leaves one with worries about reoccurrence and length of life. The fear of death after a diagnosis of cancer can override the potential loss of intimacy and sexuality. Almost half of cancer survivors report ongoing problems with sexual functioning.[3] These problems cause changes in sexual self-esteem, body image, and sexual performance.

We often think of cancer as a disease that strikes the elderly or unhealthy. However, we hear more and more about teens and young adults who have cancer. This brings up many issues that are unique to the young, such as how to get back into the dating scene and talk about the cancer and its effects, fertility issues, early hormonal changes, medical insurance, sex, and more. A very helpful book, *Everything Changes* by Kairol Rosenthal, brings the compelling stories of Rosenthal and twenty-five other cancer survivors to the reader.[4] Rosenthal provides resources, advice, wisdom, and compassion for the twenty- and thirty-something cancer survivors. In the section of the book entitled "Beyond In and Out," Rosenthal says, "Here is the secret that most people our age don't know: you can have extremely gratifying, sexy, hot, kinky, loving, romantic, and intimate relationships by touching, cuddling, kissing, and other kinds of sex that do not include penetration."[5]

There are many different types of cancer, and we will look at cancers that particularly affect sexuality. Most cancers and their treatment do affect sexual functioning, and you can find more information in the resources section about the effects of cancer on sexuality.

Women and Cancer   Cancer can have an effect on how a woman experiences herself as a sexual being. The location of the cancer may profoundly impact the woman, her sexual response, and her body image. Gynecological cancers will affect a woman's reproductive/sexual organs. Women with other types of cancer, such as colon, anal, or bladder, will also experience physical and sexual changes due to treatment and surgery results.

Breast cancer can affect sexuality on several different levels. For many women, breasts are a source of sexual pleasure and an important part of body image. Even with reconstruction of the breast, there are far-reaching emotional consequences for the woman and her partner. Alterations in sensation over the scar are common, and a woman may express that she prefers not to be touched in the area of the scar.

Chemotherapy results in profound changes to a woman's sexual self. Loss of appetite, nausea, hair loss, and fatigue can all have an overwhelming effect on body image and desire. Chemotherapy affects hormones and may lead to the cessation of ovarian activity. Most women report decreased libido, dyspareunia (pain with vaginal penetration) due to vaginal dryness, and menopausal symptoms (decrease of lubrication, hot flashes, insomnia, weight gain, etc.).

Radiation impacts sexuality because it affects energy levels, as well as local changes to the skin. Radiation to the breast can cause swelling, tenderness, and sensitivity. When radiation is focused on the pelvic area, scarring, vaginal tenderness, and inflammation can interfere with sex. Sometimes, sore spots occur in the vagina, which may take months to heal.

Rebecca, in her mid-forties, stated that following the diagnosis and treatment of her breast cancer, she felt suddenly very alone. It seemed to Rebecca that her girlfriend and family slipped quickly back into the regular routine of life and wanted her to do the same. She explained, "I'm still afraid of the cancer returning and my body is not the same, but no one seems to want to talk about it anymore. It's as though they all feel that I'm cured now and we are just supposed to pick up again where we were before the diagnosis. It's not that simple for me!"

The ability to return to a healthy view of one's sexual self depends on the capacity to find pleasure in sexual activities again, the comfort with the body after treatment, and the reaction to physical changes. If the cancer treatment affects hormone production and the reproductive system, survivors of cancer need to seek advice from a physician regarding dealing with the painful side effects of vaginal dryness and other menopausal symptoms. Vaginal moisturizers and lubricants can reduce the discomfort and may lead to a gradual resumption of sexual activity. Medication, individual therapy, support groups, and couples therapy can be helpful for the emotional needs of the couple.

How can couples cope with the sexual changes following cancer treatment? This is a time to experiment with other types of touch and arousal. Guide your partner's hand and let him or her know what your sexual turn-ons are. Sexual exploration may not end in intercourse, but there can be pleasure and intimacy that is satisfying and reassuring to both of you. See the description of sensate focus in appendix C at the end of this book.

 SEXUAL HEALING

My partner has a form of gynecological cancer and we have put sex on hold for the time being. I'm involved in her treatment and attend all her appointments with her. I want to be supportive and sensitive. I am okay with other ways of pleasing each other sexually, but I'm scared to talk to my partner. I know she's having a hard time dealing with this and I don't want to add to the problem. I'm not ready to give up on sex, either.

It's great that you are so supportive of your partner and are going with her to her appointments. She is probably struggling with her sense of self and examining how she feels about sex at this point. This is a time to connect and find out what you need as a couple to enjoy intimacy. Regarding treatment, be sure to ask questions about the side effects of any treatments, medications, and surgeries. It's hard to deal with what is unknown. Talking about sex is uncomfortable even under the best circumstances, so it may be more difficult to have a conversation about it with your partner at this time. Read this chapter with your partner, using it as a resource to encourage dialogue in this area. Seek out a support group, and we encourage your partner to do the same. Support groups can also help in the area of sex, as a way to find out how others deal with this sensitive issue. Find a certified sex therapist who can work with you on redefining your sex life. In chapter 10, we'll look at how to find a sex therapist qualified to help with your concerns. Additionally, read about treatment for sexual pain in appendix B; a urogynecological physical therapist may be able to help make sex more comfortable for your partner. There are additional suggestions in the resources section of this book.

Men and Cancer   Cancer in men, particularly testicular, prostate, colon, anal, and penile cancers, results in sexual problems. A diagnosis of one of these cancers and the treatment can affect a man's self-image and feelings of masculinity. Treatment may impact sexual functioning and can have significant side effects, including urinary incontinence, infertility, erectile dysfunction (ED), and fatigue. Psychologically, the treatment's side effects may leave a man with significantly lowered self-esteem and self-confidence.

For men with genital cancer treated with radiation, ED is common. After radiation treatment, ejaculatory disturbances often occur, such as reduction of the volume of ejaculate, absence of ejaculation, and pain with orgasm.[6] Radiation treatment for male genital cancers can cause tenderness and sensitivity to the surrounding areas. Infertility may be a concern and needs to be addressed with a health-care provider. There is more information on sexual side effects of cancer in the resources section.

When a man is diagnosed and treated for cancer, both partners are affected. Initially, the couple may find themselves drawing closer and focusing on the survival aspects of the diagnosis. Once the treatment has begun and the side effects are evident, the sexual relationship needs to be discussed. Talking about the issues of libido, ED, and possible erectile aids is no easy task. However, discussions increase intimacy and provide understanding.

> Ray and Ruth talked to their therapist about their feelings regarding the surgical side effects of Ray's prostate cancer. They both discussed feelings of loss after realizing that Ray was no longer able to have an erection. Although Ruth enjoyed her own orgasm, they both missed their previous sexual interaction that included Ray's erection and orgasm. Ray also discussed the shock he had experienced when he discovered that he had to deal with both incontinence and erectile failure.

> Permission was needed for the grieving process so feelings of sadness and loss could be thoroughly explored in therapy. Additionally, Ray was encouraged to try all forms of erectile enhancement as prescribed by his physician. Throughout therapy, Ruth became more open to exploring other forms of sexual stimulation, including the use of a vibrator and oral sex.

In time, the incontinence was no longer an issue, and Ray discovered that he could achieve an erection with a penile injection. Using this erectile aid, Ray and Ruth learned they needed to look at this as their "new normal" for sexual response and activity. They now had to plan sex, rather than be as spontaneous as they had been in the past. However, they both agreed they found that sex could still be a loving and intimate experience. They were also pleased to discover that sex remained exciting and spicy, although it required a little more creativity, communication, and planning. Ray and Ruth also were grateful they had discovered more about their sexual selves and about the varieties of sexual pleasure beyond intercourse.

The "New Normal"

When intimacy is compounded by illness, sexuality can be uncomfortable to discuss. The physically unaffected partner will be struggling with his partner's illness and may feel that exploration of his own sexual desires seems selfish. The person dealing with his illness and its treatment will likely feel a sense of loss, fear, and sadness. He may also feel a burden to return to sexuality, but be unclear about what that means. Sex, intimacy, and life as a couple have changed dramatically. Experimenting with different types of touch or techniques may be a way for a couple to grow closer. Communication about what feels good and what doesn't can be freeing for the couple. Acknowledging that there is a "new normal" is imperative; sex can't be exactly as it was in healthier times, but a couple may find affectionate, sensual ways to reconnect.

SEX AND DISABILITY

Physical disability can take many different forms, whether it's related to a spinal cord injury, cerebral palsy, a history of polio, or any number of challenges. There is much that could be covered in discussing sex and disability, but we will briefly talk about some important areas of consideration. Also see the resources section of this book for more sources of information.

Communication about sex is imperative, especially when dealing with illness. For those with physical disabilities, communication is equally, if not more important. The World Health Organization defines physical disability as a "condition of significant loss or deviation in the function or structure of the body that results in limitations of activity."[7] Sexual desire and needs don't go away when our bodies are hurt or disabled. It's essential that the disabled person be willing to discuss desires, abilities, arousal styles, weaknesses, and limitations with his or her partner.

Many factors come into play when a disabled person is sexually involved with his or her partner, such as the recentness of the disability, the severity of the disability, which body parts are affected, and feelings about body image. Paul Joannides suggests that not only is the couple prone to the same relationship conflicts as every other couple, but they also have to deal with the problems that come along with the disability.[8] There may be sexual problems, including erectile disorder, difficulty with vaginal lubrication, reduced feeling in the genitals, and difficulty with orgasm. Some people will also require assistance in order to receive effective sexual stimulation despite physical limitations.

Often a social stigma accompanies the expression of sexual needs for the disabled. According to McCabe and Talepores, the social stigma can affect sexual esteem, satisfaction, and sexual behavior among those with disabilities.[9] The severity of the disability appears to determine the impact on these aspects of sexuality, as well as the extent of depression surrounding the sexual self. McCabe and Talepores found that disabled women tended to experience sexual encounters more positively and had less depression than the disabled men had. The authors suggest that the disabled women find tenderness and sharing more important than the physical aspect of intimacy. In this study, it was found that oral sex and cuddling in the nude were important to disabled men, while deep kissing was more important to disabled women, which substantiated the finding that genital activity was less important to the disabled women.

An excellent resource for sexuality and disability is the book *The Ultimate Guide to Sex and Disability* by Miriam Kaufman, Cory Silverberg, and Fran Odette.[10] Sex toys can be very helpful in enhancing sexual experiences when dealing with a disability, as well as the practice of Tantra. Tantra is intended to reconnect the body, the mind, the heart, and the spirit with sexuality. There is more about Tantra in chapter 9. We have included a resource section with books about Tantric sex in the back of this book. The resources section also has a list of websites that are excellent sources for adult sex toys.

HOW OLD IS "TOO OLD"?

In August 2007, the *New England Journal of Medicine* surveyed 3,005 people between 57 and 85 years of age.[11] A significant number reported that they were, in fact, sexually active into their late seventies and mid-eighties! Health problems and the lack of a partner were the biggest barriers to sex, not a lack of desire! The study found that sex with a partner in the last year was reported by 73 percent of those aged 57 to 64, 53 percent of those aged 64 to 75, and 26 percent of those aged 75 to 85. Interestingly enough, of those who were sexually active, most said they were having sex at least two or three times a month. However, about half of the people surveyed reported they had a "bothersome" sexual problem, such as erectile dysfunction, low desire, difficulty with lubrication, or inability to achieve orgasm.

What makes the difference between couples who have great sex into midlife and beyond and those who don't? In his book, *Better Than Ever*, Dr. Bernie Zilbergeld reported on sexually active people age forty-five and over, using the notion of "lovers," those who reported their sex life was "good" or "wonderful"; and "non-lovers," those who did not report at least a "good" sex life.[12] Zilbergeld concluded that the two means by which these groups differed were in the areas of 1) relating to each other, and 2) their intention to have and maintain a good sex life. In other words, he found that the lovers were more likely to relate to one another with respect, acceptance, tolerance, and mutual support than were the non-lovers. Zilbergeld discovered that, sexually, the lovers were more likely than the non-lovers to have and maintain intentional sensual interaction.

What does this mean for sexual encounters after midlife? Couples need to remain playful and sensual at all ages and to make a conscious effort to stay sexually active and connected. Respect and support provide a thriving environment for couples as they age.

COMPONENTS OF OPTIMAL SEX

Kleinplatz and her colleagues give us the concept of optimal sex.[13] They define optimal sex as being different from what the media portrays as "great sex." Further, a person can experience optimal sex despite the effects of "age, illness, and disability." Based on 64 interviews with men and women (25 were between the ages of 60 and 82 and had been in relationships of 25 years or longer), Kleinplatz and her team identified the following eight characteristics as common in those who experience optimal sex:

- Sense of being present, focused, and embodied
- Connection, alignment, merger, being in sync
- Deep sexual and erotic intimacy
- Extraordinary communication, heightened empathy
- Authenticity, lack of inhibition, transparency
- Transcendence, bliss, peace, transformation, healing
- Exploration, interpersonal risk-taking, fun
- Vulnerability and surrender

Two other factors were identified as minor components:

- Intense physical sensation and orgasm (in the sense that orgasm often occurs but is not necessary)
- Lust, desire, chemistry, attraction

As we age, many physiological changes will affect us, influencing mood, self-esteem, body image, and the ability to respond sexually. Both men and women will notice physical and sexual changes as they progress through the aging process. Keep in mind that with a recipe of creativity and patience, this can be a sexually gratifying time of life with a seasoned partner.

Issues for Women

Women in their thirties, forties, and fifties may experience emotional, sexual, and physical changes associated with aging. The onset of these changes, called perimenopause, can last from two to fifteen years before a woman reaches menopause (going a year without menstruation). As a woman begins the journey through perimenopause and menopause, she may experience insomnia, mood fluctuations, difficulty concentrating, hot flashes, weight gain, and lowered libido. All of these symptoms may affect a woman's desire to be sexual.

When Diana was fifty-two, she became involved with a man whom she called "the love of [her] life." "For the first year of our relationship, I had the best sex I have ever had! No worries about getting pregnant, raising kids, or being too tired at the end of the day to 'get it on!' Almost a year to the day that we first made love, along came the hot flashes, night sweats, mood swings, and vaginal dryness. As if that wasn't enough, my fifty-nine-year-old partner began to have problems with his erections." Diana was in tears, asking her therapist if this was "some sort of cruel joke."

Estrogen levels will decline in menopause and will bring about vaginal dryness and thinning of the vaginal walls. There are positives, however! Supplemental vaginal estrogen, in the form of cream, an estrogen-containing ring, or a vaginal tablet, can be helpful for comfortable sex after menopause, as this will keep the vagina supple and moist. Many products are available to help with the physical symptoms.

Hormone replacement is not for everyone. For a woman who has had breast cancer, a family history of breast cancer, or other gynecological cancers, she will need to consider the risks and benefits of hormone replacement, even topical estrogen creams. A low dose of hormones may lessen the negative psychological and physical symptoms of menopause, but this is something that each woman will need to explore with her health-care provider.

During menopause, testosterone, the hormone of desire, decreases. On an encouraging note, Helen Fisher explains that, for middle-aged women, although estrogen decreases with menopause, testosterone becomes more dominant and able to be expressed more fully.[14] One study showed that, as a result of this chemical change, 40 percent of middle-aged women felt they weren't getting enough sex!

As a woman ages, changes in appearance may affect her body image. If body image is influencing sexual desire and self-esteem, a woman may want to discuss this with a therapist and her partner. Talking about the impact that body image has on self-esteem can lead to self-acceptance. This can be a time to get past some of the more superficial aspects of sex, and a time to discover different facets of oneself and deepen intimacy in other ways.

Many women reinvent themselves in midlife, seeking to find who they are outside of being "mom" and "partner." Midlife can be a time to examine new passions and focus, as well as try new things we didn't allow ourselves before! Take piano lessons or learn to paint. Reconnect with old friends or make new ones. Surround yourself with affirming people. Take short vacations, even alone, to relax and get reacquainted with who you are at this exciting turning point in life. Most of all, don't give up on sex! We are sexual beings, and our sexuality is part of who we are at every age.

Issues for Men

With age, one of the major physiological changes for men is that attaining an erection will take longer and require more direct penile stimulation. The erection will not be as firm, it is more likely to fade, and there is a lessened need to ejaculate at each sexual opportunity. These changes can be challenging when comparing current sexual responses to those of one's youth.

Most young males learn that their sexual response is easy, autonomous, and predictable. A man in his forties or beyond will need to learn to accept a variable response pattern and begin discussing these changes. Erectile changes can become very challenging if there is a sense of having to be "on your game" for all sexual encounters. Performance pressure can become the death knell for a satisfying sexual relationship. Appendix A contains information regarding various sexual disorders for males.

Testosterone augmentation and the use of erectile aids are issues to discuss with a health-care provider. A medical professional needs to assess and monitor the use of these aids. These medical interventions can be integrated into a sexual relationship with honesty and understanding. The use of Viagra, or one of the other erectile aids, is not an automatic answer to erectile changes. In order to have a satisfying sex life as we age, there's a need to have a more intimate and interactive lovemaking style than was realized at other life stages.

🌿 SEXUAL HEALING

I am a fifty-three-year-old man. I have had a pretty good sex life with my partner of thirty years, up until now. She thinks I don't want her any more, but the reality is that I am having difficulty getting an erection. I don't want to tell her, so I just avoid any sexual contact. I don't want her to feel bad, either. She even asked if I'm having an affair! What do I do? I feel like a failure!

First of all, read what you can about how the body changes when a man ages. You can find ideas for books in the resources section at the end of this book. How have your sexual responses changed when you masturbate? Can you achieve an erection when you self-stimulate? If so, are you doing anything differently when you masturbate than when you're with your partner? Communicating this to your partner is important, not only for you, but for your sexual relationship. It's likely you will both feel better after discussing the issue. Think about why this is difficult to talk about. For instance, is it embarrassment or feeling as though you need to fix the problem? Don't let any reason keep you from discussing this with your partner. It's pretty safe to say that she notices that something is wrong, and she may not understand what it is. She needs to know, and she needs to know how to help stimulate you sexually in order for you to achieve erection. This is a common problem as men age. Don't look at it as failure! This is a time when you can redefine your sexual experiences with your partner! The experimentation to find what works can be fun, as well as create a different sexual experience. A medical exam is also necessary in order to rule out any physical problem that may be playing a role.

※ ※ ※

In a man's twenties, orgasm and ejaculation are often the goal of sex. But as a man ages, sexual arousal and response are not so automatic, and sex may be seen as a performance instead of a pleasurable way to connect. Rather than seeing sex as a performance matter, be flexible, adopting a pleasure-oriented style to sexual encounters. The partner's role becomes very important as the sex act becomes less about "getting off," and more about the give and take of pleasure. These changes don't mean that sex is over! Far from it! This is a time of re-evaluating and renegotiating one's sexual relationship and sexual needs. This time in life can be enjoyed without being performance focused, as it was in the past.

Be creative in sexuality, focusing on intimacy and touch. Talking about sexual needs and the way that our bodies have changed can bring about a deepening of intimacy, creating a bond that allows us to experiment more freely. If communication is a struggle, read chapter 6 of this book to learn more about these issues.

MOVING ACROSS THE BRIDGE

Affirming yourself and your partner during life's challenges can be difficult, but very rewarding in terms of connecting as a couple. Remember,
life never remains the same. Change happens, and what you do with
that change can make or break your relationship. Work hard at making
it a time for change and growth with your partner instead of a time for
isolation and stagnation on your own. By not talking to your partner, the
bridge becomes broken and impassable.

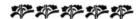

SEXERCISES

I. If you haven't already made a sex date with your partner, give it a try.
It may not feel very romantic to have to plan sex, but it's much more romantic than not having sex at all. Be creative and do something to shake
things up a bit, like a different location for sex or a new adult toy.

II. With life's changes, you may need to grieve a loss. Write in your
journal about what you see as loss and how it affects your life. It might
be a loss related to parenting, infertility, illness, aging, or physical limitations. Talk to your partner about how you feel, and listen to how your
partner feels.

III. After writing about loss, write now about any feelings of anger that
you have. It's common to feel angry about the changes that are taking
place as you age or deal with illness. Write about your feelings of frustration regarding any aches or pain, the changes in your body's tone and
appearance, the loss of function, or the inability to have sex as you did
in your youth. Talk about your feelings to your partner. You may also
need to discuss these emotions with a therapist as it can be challenging
to work through these emotions of anger.

IV. If you are on medication, talk to your health-care provider in order
to understand if sexual side effects may be an issue.

V. Redefine your sex life. Write what sex means to you during this time
in your life. How has this stage affected you? What are your expecta-

tions? What do you want from your partner? Whatever your life changes may be, think about your "new normal." What adjustments do you need to make in order to keep sex, sensuality, intimacy, or affection alive in your relationship?

VI. If you have a physical challenge with sex, answer the following questions and talk with your partner about each:

- What types of activities are important to each of you for "good" sex?
- What hurts?
- What feels good?
- Is there another way to do things?
- Is arousal painful?
- If certain types of sexual activity cause you pain, are they worth it?
- How often do you each expect to have sex?

VII. Sometimes, with painful or uncomfortable sex, we begin to make internal statements that are destructive. The following statements are common and we have included some "reframing" statements (healthier and more positive statements). Look these over, write some of your own commonly uttered statements, and try to reframe them.

1. "I feel guilty about what I am putting my partner through."
   - "This is an opportunity for my partner and me to stretch beyond our old habits of sexual behaviors and try some new things."
2. "I don't feel like having sex these days. I don't seem to have any desire now."
   - "I know that I don't feel turned on like I used to, but I can enjoy caressing, kissing, and stroking."
3. "Sex is painful."
   - "When sex is painful, I'll stop and acknowledge that I'm in control of my sexual experience. My partner and I know that if sex hurts, we can explore other sexual experiences, such as massage, cuddling, kissing, and oral and/or manual stimulation."

II

ARE YOU TALKING TO ME?

My partner and I seem to have very different expectations and desires when it comes to sex. I feel like we are becoming so distant, both emotionally and sexually.

—Male, age 40

6

DIALOGUES OF SEXUAL COMMUNICATION

Engaging Each Other

Talk about sex? Are you kidding me! I can't even get him to talk about our broken garbage disposal!

—Female, age 32

- Do you talk to your partner about your sexual relationship?
- Are you able to listen to your partner without getting upset and defensive?
- Do you have conversations with your partner about not being sexually satisfied that don't end up in a huge fight?
- Are you aware of your nonverbal communication?
- Can you and your partner share feelings that are important regarding sex?

In the very best of situations, communicating can be difficult. Add the topic of sex into the mix and you have a discussion that can be complicated and tricky. It's safe to say that most of the couples and individuals who walk into our office are having interpersonal problems of some sort, and communication plays a big part in resolving those problems. When it comes to communicating with your partner, we want you to have good, productive conversations with each other, especially regarding sex.

Chris and Carmen were having difficulty discussing the sexual differences in their relationship. Carmen was frustrated that Chris didn't seem
interested in talking about his erectile disorder and that their sex life had
become nonexistent. She also felt Chris might not be attracted to her.
Carmen finally became frustrated enough to confront Chris, saying "Why
don't you want to talk about our sexual problem? It must be something
about the way I look, since you obviously don't seem to want me and
can't stay hard!" Chris yelled back at Carmen, "Oh, right! Blame me for
everything! I guess it doesn't matter that I get too tired to talk about all of
this!" Both Chris and Carmen turned their backs on each other, both felt
misunderstood, and the problem didn't get resolved.

Expressing, listening, and communicating . . . it sounds simple, but
why is saying what we're thinking and feeling such potential for disaster?
It seems that while we heard all kinds of lectures as we were growing up,
no one sat us down and gave us the "handling conflict" talk or the "communication" talk, and we've already discussed that most of us didn't get
the "sex" talk. As a result, we have to erase some of our bad communication habits and learn better techniques in order to have our sexual needs
heard, as well as hear about our partner's needs.

SAFETY IN SHARING

When we use the communication techniques described in this chapter,
we create an environment that allows a degree of safety for both partners. Defensiveness and sharp tongues can make us feel unsafe and
insecure. It's difficult to express ourselves openly and honestly when
safety becomes compromised. In a relationship, it's up to each partner
to take care of the other partner's sense of safety, as well as their own.
If safety is a problem in the relationship, it's critical to mend the rift that
has occurred. If the rift is too massive for the techniques in this book,
see a therapist who can help you find a safe place in the relationship
before tackling difficult issues such as sex.

SEXUAL HEALING

The way my partner and I communicate is horrible! Every time we disagree, I find that my partner calls me awful names and yells at me. It's

pretty scary. Then, after the tirade is over, I'm blamed for the way my partner reacted! Sometimes I feel scared that my partner is going to hit me, but it hasn't gone that far. My friend says this is verbal abuse, but I'm just not sure it is. Is this abuse?

This does sound like verbal abuse. No one deserves to be criticized, demeaned, called names, threatened, or blamed when tension is high in their relationship. We recommend that you seek help, and encourage you to trust your "gut feelings." You may already be struggling with verbal abuse, and your fear of it turning into physical abuse is a real possibility. See a mental health provider who can help you regain control of your life and your self-esteem so you can make the choices you need in order to feel safe. Call your local domestic violence center or the domestic abuse hotline below to get more information.

Sometimes feeling unsafe becomes more than just the inability to say what we feel. If you feel as though you are in danger, the first order of business is to have a safety plan in place. If you feel there is a threat of abuse, you can call the National Domestic Violence Hotline at 1-800-799-SAFE (7233) or TTY 1-800-787-3224 for help in crisis intervention or safety planning. There is a big difference between miscommunication and abuse. No one should live in a state of fear.

COMMUNICATION 101

Throughout this chapter, there are tips to ensure that good communication about any topic is fostered and maintained. When we are in an intimate relationship, it's not unusual that conversations get heated. We may have to take a step back and remember what we are trying to achieve. As a couple, think about what the basic rules will be when sitting down to talk. These basics can be discussed ahead of time and will be in the background of all conversations, whether the context is sexual or not.

Ground Rules

Ground rules should be established and discussed ahead of time. These rules can be written down and kept handy so they can be referred to during an argument, if necessary. Talk about practical and logistical matters that are important to each partner, so these basics don't become part of the argument. For example, you might want to discuss something your partner did last night that you found to be troubling, but it might be inappropriate to bring this particular argument up to your partner in the morning when you are both rushing around and trying to get out the door! Bringing the matter up at this particular time may get a response such as, "Are you serious? Could this have possibly waited until this evening when we aren't trying to get to work?" Consider these ideas to discuss when you negotiate ground rules for any serious conversation:

- Think about the time and place you want to have serious conversations. There will always be exceptions; some issues can't wait and have to be addressed immediately. However, most problems can wait several hours in order to make the environment more optimal for sharing your concerns. It may make it easier to talk if you choose a time after the dinner dishes are put away and the dogs have been fed.
- Agree about how to take a time-out. Generally, one partner might say something like, "I really want to resolve this issue, but I'm having difficulty hearing you right now and need some time to process this. Let's take a break and come back to the discussion after dinner."
- Discuss the people with whom you can and can't talk to about the issue. Everyone needs a support system, so try to be fair. Respect each partner's desire to keep certain people out of your issues. For instance, you may not want your partner to discuss your relationship problems with your mother or the neighbor down the street who likes to gossip.
- Keep in mind that you love this person and you both have the same goal, which is to have the best relationship possible. Remember to be kind to each other.
- You won't always agree with everything your partner says. It's okay to disagree, but again, be kind. We all have different points of view and deserve to express them with respect and be heard with respect.

This step of establishing ground rules is very important, and it should be discussed as soon as possible. It helps us create a sturdy foundation that we can base future disagreements on. We can't change the way we have communicated in the past, but we can move forward with better skills for handling the way we talk to each other.

Nonverbal Communication

Verbal communication and nonverbal communication are the ways we express ourselves to others. So far, we have only been discussing the verbal ways that we communicate with each other, which is what we articulate or verbalize to the other person. Nonverbal communication, on the other hand, is a little more complicated and can be a look, tone of voice, volume, the way we present our bodies, or our proximity to others. It's been estimated that over 90 percent of a message's impact is nonverbal (this includes vocal intonation and body movements).

Body language and facial expressions can be misunderstood, and if we don't address the issue, nonverbal communication can cause problems. At times, we may assume something after we see our partner turn his head away, roll his eyes, or clench his jaw. We might misperceive a tone of voice or lack of response. If we get a particular message through nonverbal means, we need to be sure to get verbal clarification from the other person. As individuals, we should take responsibility for the unspoken messages that we convey with our own body language.

 SEXUAL HEALING

My partner often gives me "the look" or uses a mean tone of voice instead of telling me what I've done wrong. I get very frustrated, because I can't read my partner's mind, and I just want to know what the problem is! How can I get to the bottom of this?

This is a great question. We can really get bogged down when it comes to body language, and since it is nonverbal, the problem is often not discussed. I'm glad to hear you want to address it! When your partner gives you a look or uses a certain tone of voice, try to talk about it right away. You can say something like, "Just now, you gave me a look and it seems like I've upset you. Can we talk about what's bothering you?" If you say it in a way that can be received, it will create a safe environment to discuss the problem.

PROBLEMS IN COMMUNICATION

Now that we have some basic rules and a foundation to build upon, let's look at some of the problems that occur in relationships that result from the way we communicate with each other. Some of these problems can be resolved easily, while some will take more effort. Regardless, when we deal with these problems effectively, it opens a door to the possibility of growth and connectedness in our relationship.

Common Communication Blunders

There are times when we talk to each other and the words just don't seem to come out right or the interpretation of the words is "off kilter." We call these "communication blunders" and they can have a damaging effect on conversations with our partner. Communication blunders often result in fights with no resolution. The problem with each of these blunders is that defenses go up and no one feels heard or validated. When communicating in a negative manner, it's usually at the expense of the partner *and* the relationship. Here are examples of common communication blunders that can affect a relationship, both in and out of the bedroom.

Communication Blunders
Making Assumptions
"No, that's not what I said! Why do you put words in my mouth?"

Making assumptions about what the other person wants or what the other person is saying is a common communication blunder. We often interpret our partner's feelings and assume that we know what they are saying without checking with them first. Consider this response instead:

*"I hear what you are saying, and it sounds like you heard _____.
I'm sorry it came across that way. That must feel _____ (i.e., disappointing, annoying, frustrating)."*

Remember to take responsibility for your part in the misunderstanding. Admitting that you might have come across in a way you didn't intend will go a long way in resolving miscommunication.

Defensiveness

"You're blaming me for our lack of sex! But you come home so late from work and watch TV all the time!"

You can go back and forth, giving each other a laundry list of ways you have each "messed up," but nothing will be resolved. Here's a better idea:

"It sounds like you're feeling frustrated and ignored. Let's talk about how we can find time for each other."

Sometimes validation is all your partner needs to be able to move on from the situation. You both feel closer because you are listening to why your partner is upset.

The Silent Treatment

"Fine! I won't talk to you then! Just leave me alone!"

The silent treatment! Have you ever done this or been on the receiving end of it? The silent treatment is a hostile way of handling anger. Nothing gets resolved and it can go on for days! When the silent treatment goes on for a period of time, it gets harder and harder to get out of the "hostility trap" that has been created. You want to get to a resolution, and the silence is counterproductive. Begin a more constructive dialogue that will help you get past the silence. Try this:

"I feel sad about our arguing, and I don't want us to just shut each other out. Let's go out on the porch and talk about one of our tough issues, right after dinner."

Couples often put up walls to each other over the course of time. Differences, hurts, and boredom take their toll and we find that we're distant roommates. Begin the dialogue with one topic of concern and really practice listening to your partner.

"Old Baggage" in the Trunk

"I'm so sick of the way you talk to me! You make me feel like I can't do anything right! You're just like my dad! No wonder we're not having sex very often!"

Sounds like old baggage is triggered in this remark. Think about the feelings that come up when you hear your partner talk to you, and remember times in the past when you may have felt this way. When you detect the old familiar feelings from your past creeping up, deal with them as soon as possible. How can you express them better?

"The feeling I'm having right now reminds me of how I used to feel when my dad criticized me. Let's back up and talk about things."

Be aware that your "hot button" issues may have to do with your own past. Your partner may not even realize the emotional impact of his or her statements.

Making Threats
"I'm sick of the way you treat me! I'm outta here!"

It's hard for you as a couple to resolve a problem when your relationship is threatened in this manner. Sometimes we feel so discouraged about our communication or our relationship that we just want out, but constant threats to leave undermine the relationship. What would be a less threatening statement?

"I feel scared that we are growing farther apart. When I feel scared like this, I tend to withdraw. But I love you and we've built a life together. Let's talk about this issue."

Threats to leave a relationship are never productive. Take time-outs when you need them, but come back to troubling issues after you've had time to cool off.

The above communication blunders are common, but even so, destructive. They take their toll on your relationship and, thus, your sex life. Good communication promotes connectedness, but when you aren't connected, it can seem like your partner is speaking a foreign language. A lack of connection can affect every part of a relationship, especially sexual encounters.

"The Blame Game"

It's been our experience in private practice that one of the partners in a relationship often comes to us with an agenda. The partner makes the appointment (or tells their partner to call, "or else!") and seems to have the intention of telling his or her side of the story, hoping the therapist will agree that the partner is at fault, passing judgment, and the partner will then have to realize they are "wrong." Then it is our job as therapists to "fix" the other person. What a surprise when we actually begin discussing "the couple" as being the problem, and not "the person" as the problem!

When the argument boils down to who is to blame, it pits the couple against each other. In a relationship, the goal is to work together, as a team, instead of going "head to head." It's easy for couples to forget their partner is the person they want to be with on a daily basis and spend their life with, the person they love. So, how do couples get around the "blame" problem? When this is an issue in a relationship, it's important to consider thinking about one's partner in a different way.

As therapists, we ask the couple to think of speaking to their partner in a way that makes the partner feel safe and validated. Many couples have trouble with this, as each person doesn't seem to understand why he or she has to change. After all, if the other person would only come around, everything would be "fine."

Very often, we tell people in therapy that "you can't change or control your partner, but you can change or control the reactions you have to the partner or the situation." Suggestions can be made, but changing the partner or the way the partner interacts is never an option. This doesn't mean "giving in," or compromising one's feelings or values, but becoming "allies." By becoming allies, we can respect our partner's needs and emotional well-being while working on getting our own needs met. If we want change in the way we interact as a couple, we have to try individually to make a change in the way we interact with our partner.

Anger and Venting

When we say angry words without considering the other person's feelings, nothing gets resolved. We should never feel as though we have to walk on eggshells around someone we care about, but we do have to take a moment to calm down and consider how we're going to get our point across and be heard by our partner. If we aren't being heard, then our feelings get buried, only to resurface at another time. No one benefits when we simply sling around the other person's shortcomings.

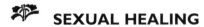 SEXUAL HEALING

My partner and I had a huge fight and we ended up saying terrible things to each other. This always happens when we have an issue. It seems we never get past tearing each other down. What do we do?

You may have been told since you were a child that you should express your anger when you're mad. This is true, but "expressing your anger" is not all there is to it. Simply throwing your anger at someone allows you to walk away feeling better. But what about the other person? When you express anger with someone you care about, consider the other person and their feelings, even though you are upset. You want to be treated with respect and tender loving care, so the best way to get it is to give it. Think about what you're angry about and express it in a way that isn't just vomiting venom all over your partner.

❀❀ ❀❀ ❀❀

It isn't always easy to simply feel anger, think about it, and express it in a kind way to one's partner. Many times, we allow the anger to build up inside, and, before we know it, there are other angry events piled up on top. When the anger finally "blows," it's a nasty mess that ends up being hurtful and out of control. Of course, the best thing to do is deal with each angry incident so that it doesn't get to the "blowing" point, but that's easier said than done.

If you feel you can't discuss anger with your partner without blowing up, there are ways that anger can be defused so you can talk about it in a more rational way. One way you can do this is to try writing a letter to the person to whom the anger is directed, no holds barred. This means writing a letter that allows you to express the brunt of your anger, in any words or tone necessary. This is not something you want anyone to see, as it could be hurtful to the other person. The purpose is to let off some steam, so that when you do express the anger to the other person, the message has been toned down a bit. If you're in therapy, it might be helpful to take the letter with you to a session to discuss its meaning and the depth of your hurt or anger with the therapist. Again, it's best to then destroy the letter.

Other ways to defuse anger are to talk about your feelings with a close trusted friend, exert energy with exercise, write in a journal, or express yourself creatively.

Experience and Perception

Perception plays a big part in how we communicate with others; specifically, how we interpret situations. Misperception can occur due to many factors, such as our own baggage, past experiences, societal attitudes, religious beliefs, and a whole realm of other variables. Every person has a different perception, as each of us has a different experience of life. When we expect someone to see the world as we see it, we end up disappointed and angry, while the other person feels misunderstood.

Differences in perception can wreak a lot of havoc, but it's worthwhile to try to understand why the people in our lives see the world the way they do. The way to do this is to ask them and listen to the way they perceive situations and events, not just assuming or putting words in the other person's mouth. When we fail to listen or ask for clarification, we are actually seeing the world through our *own* experience and perception, and not trying to see it through someone else's eyes. Communication and listening are ways to connect to other people, but they have to be deliberate and heartfelt. When the other person feels as though we are interested in hearing his or her perception and trying to understand, it can make the difference between feeling acknowledged and feeling lonely.

BETTER WAYS TO COMMUNICATE

Many communication techniques can bring couples together and help them feel heard by one another. Let's examine several ways to improve communication and enhance the relationship.

Saying the Words in a Way That Can Be Heard

Marissa and Martin came to therapy due to communication problems in their relationship. Marissa was upset because there were some sexual problems that she felt they should address. Martin felt that if they would just calm down and treat each other better, the problem would go away.

During the therapy session, Marissa stated, "You are always making excuses about sex! I can't even talk to you about it!" Martin got defensive and shouted back, "Maybe your attitude is the problem! Why would I even want to talk to you?" Working with the couple on this particular conversation, the therapist pointed out that when Marissa was pointing fingers, Martin was not able to receive her words. The therapist went on to explain that, by all means, Marissa should talk about the issue, but asked Marissa what she thought would help in order for Martin to hear what she was saying and not become defensive. The therapist asked Marissa to try to rephrase the words. Marissa said, "I feel as though our sex life is struggling. What can we do to help each other get our needs met?" Martin was able to hear and receive what Marissa was saying. Martin responded by asking what Marissa thought they were struggling with in their sex life. They were finally on the right track to getting both of their needs met.

How did Marissa change the conversation? First, she made Martin her ally instead of an enemy by stating the issue as a "we" problem, instead of a "you" problem. Second, Marissa refrained from pointing fingers. As a result, Martin was better able to understand the specific problem that was bothering Marissa rather than getting caught up in her emotions.

Paraphrasing

Paraphrasing is a technique used to allow a person to repeat back what was heard and get clarification regarding the meaning of the words. For instance, we might say, "Why don't you help me with the housework? It seems like I do everything around here!" The other person would then paraphrase by repeating the thought back in his or her own words. "I hear you saying that you would like me to help around the house more, so you don't feel like you are doing all the housework." Then, we can either acknowledge understanding or state again the message we were trying to communicate. Paraphrasing is important because it gives a couple the opportunity to be sure each person is expressing what they want to say correctly, but even more importantly, that he or she is being *heard* correctly. Let's look at an example of a communication misunderstanding.

Stan was upset and approached his partner, saying, "Why is it that we don't have sex very often? It seems like we hardly ever have time for each other." His partner, taking his words personally, spouted back by saying, "All you care about is sex! I guess you don't think I have anything else to do other than pleasure you!" Stan then yelled back, "Why are you making this about you? Can't we just have a civilized conversation?"

Let's try this conversation again using the technique of paraphrasing.

Stan says, "Why is it that we don't have sex very often? It seems like we hardly ever have time for each other." By paraphrasing, his partner might say, "Sounds like you think we don't have sex very often and we don't have time for each other." Stan can then say, "Yes, that is exactly what I'm thinking." In this case, Stan feels heard and the couple can continue to discuss the problem without defensiveness.

Try paraphrasing before taking what was said in a statement personally, which generally causes misunderstanding. Many times, it's not a personal issue, but it's someone feeling as though not all is right in the world. Let's talk a little more about this.

Use "I Feel" Statements

There is good reason why everyone from Dr. Phil to "Dear Abby" suggests that we use statements that begin with "I feel" when communicating. Because it's good, sound advice! Our feelings are a component of ourselves that generally can't be fought about, as no one can argue that we don't feel the way we do. For instance, if we say, "I don't *think* you want to be with me sexually anymore." The other person may comment, "No, you're wrong. I do want to be with you." On the other hand, it's more helpful to say, "I *feel* sad that we don't connect sexually as much as I would like." Using this type of sentence allows our partner to hear our idea more readily and it opens up a discussion. It can't be argued that a person is sad or that a person would like to connect more often. "I feel" statements sound like, "I feel _____ when _____." So, an "I feel" statement might be, "I feel worried that you're going to leave me when I come too soon."

Be Quiet and Listen!

As individuals, we often focus on getting our desires across to our partner so that we can get our needs met. What about when our partner has the need to express feelings? Sometimes our partner might bring up a problem and we focus on our own feelings rather than hearing what our partner is trying to get across to us. How do we let go of our own feelings for a moment in order to hear our partner's concerns?

1. People need to be heard when they talk. This doesn't mean simply sitting quietly and nodding occasionally! It means actively listening, trying to understand, and putting oneself in the other person's shoes.

2. Asking questions can help us to understand the other person's view more fully. When asking questions of our partner, we should ask open-ended questions, such as, "How are you feeling about our sexual relationship?" This would be a better question than "Aren't you happy with our sexual relationship?" which only requires a "yes" or "no" answer.

3. It's helpful to repeat back to the person a summary of what was heard, letting the person know we are listening and that we care about what they said. "It sounds like you feel frustrated because we don't have much time to relax and connect emotionally. Is that what you're feeling? I know I'd like to have more time to just sit out on the porch and talk, like we used to do."

4. Try validating someone's feelings instead of arguing. This doesn't mean selling yourself out. It means saying, "I hear what you're saying, and I acknowledge that you feel that way." For example, one partner might say, "We don't have sex anymore." The other partner might be tempted to respond with "Yes we do! You just want it all the time! I'm exhausted and that's the last thing on my mind these days!" Instead, you might try this response, "Sounds like you miss having sex." You can take it even further if you say, "Do you have any thoughts on how we might make more time for each other?"

5. Empathic listening is listening to a partner's heart with our own heart. Empathy is the ability to imagine oneself in another's situation and understand the other's desires, ideas, feelings, and actions. For example, our partner may say, "I hate the fact that you've used porn compulsively in our relationship!" If we are being empathic, we might respond by saying, "You must feel rejected by my constant porn use. I understand why you would feel that

I might be comparing you to these images." This is an empathic answer instead of the defensive responses we may be used to hearing. It might have been tempting to say, "Do you have to nag me about my porn use when we've talked about it and it's in the past?" Empathy is a way of letting a partner know, not only that she is heard, but that the emotions behind her words are understood.

SEXUAL HEALING

My partner and I keep having fights that lead back to the same issue repeatedly. I'm tired of the same problem creeping back into everything we discuss! How many times do I have to keep discussing the same thing? How can I get my partner to quit bringing up this issue?

What a common occurrence this is! The reason this issue keeps coming back is that it's unresolved. Very often, when we are still hurting from a wound, we can move on for a time, but it keeps popping back into our lives. For instance, if the issue is that your partner feels ignored by you, the argument might begin with an accusation that you're not helping around the house and circle back around to the fact that your partner feels ignored. For whatever reason, your partner is not feeling heard about the issue.

Try discussing the issue when "the iron is cold," and not when tension is high and the conversation is heated. Bring the issue up when you are both in a good place and tell your partner you feel the problem is unresolved and you would like to work toward resolving the situation.

Use some of the listening techniques above to allow yourself to pay attention and hear what your partner is trying to say. You may be thinking, "Why do I want to bring the subject up when we are getting along just fine and it always causes a problem when we discuss it?" The bottom line is that it is a problem, and it will continue to be one until there's understanding. Resolution may come when you don't take the issue personally, but instead listen patiently, acknowledge your partner's feelings, and respond with empathy.

Disclosure—Deepening the Way We Communicate

In most long-term relationships, the conversation often goes down the same road—bills, kids, dinner, and so on. Everyday life seems to keep our conversations on the surface. What does a deeper conversation look like? Deeper ways of communicating require that we take risks, allowing our partner to know something about us that we aren't always comfortable sharing. Although disclosure is difficult, it helps to bring a couple closer. Disclosure doesn't always mean that we simply talk about an event or a particular characteristic of ourselves, although those things definitely fit the bill. Disclosure can be talking about feelings that make us raw and vulnerable, or fantasies that can be difficult to share.

The relationship deepens when one person discloses something, and then the listener receives the disclosure in a respectful, kind way. It's comforting to know that we can share something that makes us vulnerable and the information is handled with tenderness by the other person. Hearing a disclosure respectfully means that we treasure it, even if we don't necessarily agree with what is said. There is no arguing about the disclosure or correction by our partner. It simply is what it is and we accept it, treating it with care. The key here is protecting our partner's disclosure.

Reinforcing the Positive

Lacy came to therapy with her partner Larry. Lacy was upset because it seemed that conversations that Larry brought up always accentuated the negative aspects of their relationship. "It would be nice to hear just one thing that Larry thinks I do right! I feel down on myself all the time because it seems like there isn't anything good about our relationship!" Larry thought the relationship had problems, but for the most part was in love with Lacy and wanted to "get on the right track." With a little prompting, Larry was able to point out the good things about the relationship, making Lacy feel better about working on the issues that needed attention.

As couples, sometimes we focus so much on the needs that *aren't* being met that we forget to communicate to each other the needs that *are* getting met. We need to tell our partner when we are getting something from him or her that is important to us. There's no better way to get someone to repeat a behavior than acknowledging and praising what he or she has done well. It gets tiring to be in a relationship where only the negatives are being focused on, while the positive aspects are taken for granted. When having conversations about sex or any other topic, we must be sure to remind each other of the strengths regarding that topic, not just the weaknesses. Who doesn't like to hear, "That was great! I loved it when you _____"?

The Value of the Written Word

Sometimes we suggest that our clients write their feelings, keep a diary, or jot down their thoughts throughout the day. At times, we find that people have a gift for writing and can express themselves with more clarity and honesty in the written word than the spoken word. In these cases, it's a good idea to turn to this mode of communication to express feelings, dreams, desires, wounds, and hopes. One client stated, "I get to the point that talking things over with my partner is pointless. I just need some time to think, put my feelings onto paper, then rewrite, and give this to my partner. It seems to come out more clearly and so much gentler this way. Then we seem to be able to sit down and discuss things with more trust and safety."

Sometimes You Need a Line Judge

At times, communication problems overwhelm us. One of the advantages of couples therapy is that the therapist is able to observe the verbal and nonverbal communication while the couple talks and listens to each other. At times, it's a little like watching a tennis match. Couples sit in the therapist's office and appear to be opponents across the net from one another. Verbal barbs are hit back and forth. Someone drives the message down the line, causing the "opponent" to lose that point. The therapist can see one "player" get in position to put some spin on the ball and surprise their "opponent" with a response that catches them off balance. As therapists, we are in a unique position to see the eye-rolling, the shocked look of hurt, the contempt, or the longing as one partner listens to the other. We can also hear the details of each person's concerns as he or she struggles to make sense of their own feelings and be heard by their partner. It's very helpful to have that third party to make observations and give feedback.

Still using the tennis match metaphor, we like to encourage couples to become a "doubles team." In this scenario, both partners are on the same side, talking with each other, planning strategies, and encouraging one another.

COMMUNICATING LOVE TO YOUR PARTNER

 SEXUAL HEALING

My partner thinks I'm being ridiculous when I tell her I don't feel like she loves me. She tells me she's tired of having to reassure me all the time. She says I should just look at all the things she does for me. I hear what she's saying, and she does do a lot for me, but there's no affection in our relationship. I really need affection from her. What can I do?

We all have different needs when it comes to feeling loved. It sounds like affection is important to you, but your partner shows you love by doing little things for you. More than likely, neither of you are getting your "love needs" met. Generally, we show people love in a way that makes us feel loved; because that's the only way we know to express it. Just because a tender touch melts your heart doesn't mean that is the way to move your partner.

We all experience the feeling of love in different ways. What helps a person to feel loved? For some people, it's an expression of kindness or a loving word. For others, it's a touch or a physical expression. Our inclination is to show our feelings for someone else based on what makes us feel good. Is it a shoulder massage when feeling tense? An offer to help with the dishes? Flowers at work? Not only should we know what makes us feel loved, but we also need to address our partner's way of feeling loved.

PILLOW TALK

How does all this relate to sex? In previous chapters, you were challenged to think about what you have been taught about sex and your past sexual experiences, as well as issues that might affect your sex life. Our hope is that after reading the material and working through the sexercises, you are able to understand that the conversations you have with your partner about sex are sifted through many different filters. These filters include what we learned in childhood, shame, illness, differences, and many other factors that all add up to our own perceptions.

Accepting that we all carry along these "packed suitcases" can help set the stage for sexual communication.

Difficult Sexual Discussions

Here are some suggestions that might get the more difficult sexual conversations started on the right track:

- Stay out of the bedroom when you're discussing sexual problems.
- Keep your anatomy terminology neutrally charged. If you don't agree on terminology, just use correct terms to describe genitals and sex acts (vagina, penis, intercourse).
- What sexual terms are off limits? Decide this with your partner and be respectful of each other in this regard.
- Agree to stay away from shaming or demeaning each other. If one of you shares a sexual need or fantasy, be respectful, even if you have no intention of doing what is being suggested.
- Be as specific as you can, giving examples of what you are talking about and offering different options for solutions that can be discussed (with the understanding that these options can be negotiated and compromised on).
- Remind each other in the beginning of the conversation that you are both seeking a good sexual relationship and care about each other.

All the techniques that have been discussed in this chapter can be applied to a conversation about sex. Keep in mind that what your partner perceives may not be what you are actually trying to convey. Be patient and help your partner understand what you are trying to say, paying particular attention to clearing up misunderstandings. Likewise, give your partner the respect of asking clarifying questions that might help you understand the problem more fully.

"Touch Me There"

Not all sexual conversations deal with conflict. Sometimes we want to talk about our sexual feelings or better ways to get our sexual needs met, but we're embarrassed or can't find the right words. If you have been in a relationship for a while and have never verbalized your sexual desires, this may be difficult to do. How do you get across to your partner that you want something different? Let's look at some examples of ways to approach different situations using some of the communication techniques we've learned:

- You want your partner to touch you in a gentler way in the beginning of foreplay. How can you say this effectively? Start with what your partner does that turns you on—"I really love it when you touch me there, and I would love it even more if you would begin by touching me lightly! That would really turn me on!" This will get better results from your partner than telling him or her that they are touching you wrong.
- You want to discuss with your partner that you want more oral sex. How can you ask for it in a way that makes it more likely to happen? How about, "I really love to give and receive oral sex with you and it seems like we've kind of gotten away from that lately. How can we put more of that into our sex life?"
- Let's say you want to try a toy to liven things up a bit. What would be a good way to ask your partner? "I found this great website that has different lovemaking toys. After dinner, how about if we look around on the website to see if there's anything interesting?" (By the way, see the resources section for websites that sell sex toys.)
- What if your partner gets "down and dirty" too quickly? How can you ask him or her to slow it down? Try this, giving your partner a little nuzzle first, "I love when we make love to each other! I'm feeling like the experience goes pretty fast, though. What can we do to slow things down a bit?"

Remember to begin with what you like about your sex life, and then express the problem, ending with "what can *we* do to make it better?" This helps your partner know that you enjoy your sex life and you aren't pointing fingers.

Sexy-ing Up the Conversation!   Now, let's look at some fun ways to communicate differently about sex!

Secret Meanings   Think up phrases with your partner that might have different sexual meanings. Instead of saying, "Do you want to have sex?" your partner can use another phrase, like "Do we have any dessert at home?" It'll be fun to be in a group of people and hear your partner say to the group, "Have you seen any good movies lately?" The other people in the group may think he's trying to start a conversation, but you know that he really wants you to think about going home for an erotic night of passionate sex! Saying a sentence such as "The weather has been really great today" might be a clue to your partner that you have no panties on and you're ready for action!

Silent Treatment   Put a new spin on the term and make a date to seduce each other silently. Use only body language to express what you want from your partner, being sure to prolong foreplay to make it even more interesting. Make sure you practice your favorite "come hither" look first!

Kiss and Tell   Try kissing your partner's body from head to toe, describing aloud each part of your partner's body and what you love about that part. Don't stop until every part has been described! Then switch places and let your partner describe your body.

Phone Sex   If you and your partner have to be away from each other, pick up the phone! Describe what you want to do to each other and how you want to do it. Talk about how you are pleasuring yourself at that moment, and what you wish your partner was doing at that time.

"Fantasy"tic!   Sharing fantasies that we are comfortable talking about is a fun way to communicate about sex. Remember that we don't have to act on these fantasies, it's merely conversation. However, what happens between two consensual partners can be hot and sexy!

MOVING ACROSS THE BRIDGE

Good sex in a relationship depends on effective communication. Without successful communication, both verbal and nonverbal, you will likely find distance and disconnection in the bedroom. You may not have been taught valuable communication skills in your upbringing, but it's never too late to learn how to express your needs and desires. Good communication helps deepen a relationship.

🌿 🌿 🌿 🌿 🌿

SEXERCISES

I. Set a time, maybe once or twice a week, when you have a conversation together. Decide on how long each of you will talk. Begin with benign topics, limiting the conversation to about fifteen minutes, at first. If you have trouble coming up with topics, try picking a magazine or newspaper article, then discuss the points of the article. You may want to begin with topics that you tend to see eye-to-eye about, then move to more difficult subject matter. Be sure to take turns talking, dividing the time so you each get a chance to have a say.

II. In chapter 1, you wrote in your journal about safety rules. Go back to those rules and review them with your partner. Do they still fit the bill? Do you need to establish a signal for time-out? Do you need to set a specific time to come back to a particularly difficult conversation? How can your partner ensure that he or she is helping you to feel safe? Now, ask your partner the same questions. Discuss times when you have both felt unsafe. Talk about things that you could do differently to be sure that safety won't be compromised in the future.

III. Practice "I feel" statements. Each of you can come up with a statement, and the partner changes the sentence into "I feel _____ when _____."

For example, "It seems like you need to be drunk to have sex with me. You usually have a couple of glasses of wine before we have sex." Changed to "I feel worried that you've usually had several drinks when we have sex. Can we talk about this?"

For example, "You never initiate sex! What's wrong with you?" Changed to "I feel pressured to be in control of our sex life, as far as the frequency goes. It seems like I usually initiate sex. How can we deal with this?"

IV. Talk about what it would be like to disclose deeper content in your relationship. Before actually disclosing, talk about what the ground rules will be and what your expectations are after disclosing. Discuss your hesitation and concerns. Deeper conversations might include:

- Goals for the future
- Hopes you had as a child
- Happy times, sad times, frustrating times, exhilarating times . . .
- Sexual fantasies

V. Take a moment to write in your journal about a time when you felt loved and honored by your partner. How about when you were younger? What made you feel loved then? Think about what your partner did that gave you that warm, loved feeling. Ask your partner how she feels she expresses her love for you. Now, have your partner do the same thing. Are you expressing love in a way that your partner feels your love? Is your partner expressing love in a way that you feel loved?

VI. Read a book of fantasies or erotica together. Get more comfortable using sexual types of language and describing body parts. Talk about what turns you on, as well as what turns you off. Listen to your partner describe turn-ons and turn-offs. Remember, fantasies are just fantasies. Just because you talk about them doesn't mean that you have to act them out. Some are never going to be realized, but some could be fun and add spice to your relationship. You'll find more about spicing it up in chapter 9.

7

MESSAGES OF EXPECTATIONS

Expressing Your Needs

I keep thinking that, if we could just get along better, not argue so much, our sex life would improve.

—Male, age 33

- Are you and your partner having hurtful arguments about what is or is not going on in the bedroom?
- Are you concerned about your fantasies and what they might mean about you and your desire?
- Do you find yourself defending your expectations about sex?
- Are you wondering why your partner's sexual needs have changed so much over time?

Most sexual relationships begin when there is strong emotional, physical, and sensual attraction. For many of us, sex initially is frequent, spontaneous, adventurous, and passionate, followed eventually by a decline in sexual intensity. As we examined in chapter 1, this diminishing sexual desire in a long-term relationship is, in part, due to the dopamine-drenched neurological system becoming familiarized to the relationship.

Seth and Sandy talked, in therapy, about the loss they both felt recently due to the infrequency of sex and their lackluster sexual experiences. They had been together for twenty years, had two teenagers now, and were both working outside the home. Seth talked to Sandy about the initial stage of their relationship and the changes that had occurred, "You were so horny back then, and I loved it, Sandy! It was as if you couldn't get enough of me! I remember we'd have sex several times a day on the weekends, and we would call each other up with sexy phone calls at work, anticipating the sex later that afternoon or night. I know we're not as young as we were then; I've put on some weight; my hair is thinning; and you complain that you're too tired. I just miss that time so much! I've been thinking that maybe my technique isn't turning you on now or you're falling out of love with me."

Sandy assured Seth that she loved him, and she agreed that she missed their passion. She explained to Seth that she was hoping this was a temporary stage and that things might improve when the kids went to college. She said, "I'm finding that we hardly touch and it's difficult to think about sex when we're so distant. I wish I had that desire to have sex that I used to feel. It makes me sad to think that this is what we've become, just two middle-aged roommates."

It's common for couples to struggle with the changes that occur in the relationship brought on by familiarity, boredom, age, fatigue, stress, or any number of problems. Sexual and relationship challenges often bring misunderstandings, hurt, and misinterpretations. Only very fortunate couples avoid falling into the traps of unrealistic expectations or mistaken assumptions when it comes to sexual needs. Let's examine some common expectations that carry a great deal of weight for most individuals and couples: sex should be frequent; real sex is intercourse; good sex should be mind-blowing every time; orgasms should come easily if you know what to do; and sex should be spontaneous.

Assumptions also get most of us into trouble! The following mistaken assumptions will be explored: fantasies are dangerous; low desire means you need to take testosterone; if you don't orgasm, there's something wrong; low desire means there's something wrong in the relationship; if you fix the relationship, you'll fix the sexual problems; everyone's having good sex but us; and this is just a phase—our sex life will improve in time.

COMMON UNREALISTIC EXPECTATIONS

Sex Should Be Frequent

Sexual frequency is an often-debated concept. Some lucky couples share similar patterns of desire; they seem to agree on the timing and regularity of sex. However, this is the rare couple! More often, we see couples who will attempt to negotiate an agreed-upon rate of recurrence for this once passion-driven spontaneous activity. It even *sounds* boring . . . negotiations, rate of recurrence, schedules . . .

Then what's "normal frequency"? This is certainly debatable, especially when considering sexual activity other than intercourse. It appears that married or cohabitating couples vary on intercourse frequency, depending on age and years together. Two or three times per week or a few times per month is about average, according to the largest study in the United States.[1] There is no clear agreement among the experts as to what constitutes an abnormally high or abnormally low sexual appetite. However, it's understandable that tension may build when partners differ in their sexual needs and drives.

SEXUAL HEALING

My partner and I have been together for about three years now. At the beginning of our relationship, we had sex a lot and I really loved it. I'm able to orgasm pretty easily, I like a lot of variety, and I'm a really sensual person. The problem is that, for about the last year, my sex drive has lessened just a tiny bit. I mean, I'd still like to have sex about twice a week or several times on the weekend. But my partner is worried that something's wrong and he wants me to agree to have sex every day or at least every other day. I don't even feel sexy now; I feel so pressured! The fun seems to be gone. What do we do?

How frustrating for you! You're a fortunate woman to have discovered that you enjoy sex and that you're easily turned on. However, your partner's insistence that you be on a sexual schedule makes it difficult to feel the build-up of that all-important sexual energy. It sounds like the intrigue, unpredictability, and passion are squelched by his request for regularity and a high degree of frequency. It would be great if you would talk to him about all of this. Assure him of your continued attraction to him. Let him know that you still want to have sex and that you desire him as much as you did at the beginning of your relationship. Explain that you need time to simmer—you need to anticipate sex. Talk to him about engaging in many other sexual activities in order to keep the stimulation and anticipation alive—take showers together, massage one

*another, keep touching, buy some new toys, read erotica, and rediscover
some sexy fun together!*

❀ ❀ ❀

Some couples will have weeks and even months pass with little touching and no sex. Awkwardness and self-consciousness develop when
there's too much time between sexual encounters. It's much better to
continue touching and to plan sexual dates so that the disconnection
doesn't become the norm. This is one of those areas that always requires
an open discussion. Who initiates and how often can become the hid-
den power struggle that goes on for years with no one voicing the obvious—what does each person want and how often? However, intercourse
is only one type of sexual activity, and this leads to the next common
unrealistic expectation.

Real Sex Is Intercourse

Intercourse has been viewed by many to be the only legitimate definition of sex. However, this definition certainly leaves gay, lesbian, and
transsexual people marginalized as sexual couples. Additionally, when
sex equals intercourse alone, intercourse becomes the ultimate goal;
sometimes that goal isn't an attainable objective, and it's certainly not
always the sexiest or spiciest element of the interaction.

It's freeing to think of sex in its entirety: all the playful, exploratory,
varied, juicy fun that goes on before, during, and after intercourse. Penis-in-the-vagina (PIV) sex may not even be included. This notion can
be liberating for us to accept! It's an important concept to embrace because it invites relaxation, mindfulness, and acceptance into the sexual
experience. When sexual play is the emphasis, rather than orgasm or
intercourse, anxiety related to performance diminishes.

The aging process, medications, and illness will often usher in the
need for acceptance of varied sex play and not exclusively intercourse-
focused sex alone. It's essential to be open to changes in sexual desire
and arousal, ease of physical movement, energy levels, and other factors
related to the challenges of health and life stages. However, even young,
healthy people need to explore the notion that intercourse as a singular
goal will likely set them up for disappointment, failure, and boredom in
the bedroom. Therefore, younger couples would be wise to stay open

to other types of sexual scenarios, not limiting their sexual interaction to only PIV.

Since we're using initials (PIV), we want to share one of our favorites from the Bermans' book, *For Women Only*.[2] VENIS: Very Erotic Non-Insertive Sex! This includes all the other ways to be sexually connected besides intercourse. Oral touch, manual touch, rubbing, toys, and so on. So, next time you text someone, you could try, "BTW . . . VENIS . . . OMG!"

 ## SEXUAL HEALING

My partner doesn't really know what I'm dealing with because I'm embarrassed about it. I seem to be able to have an erection, but can't get to orgasm. I can get hard, penetrate, and then I go and go and . . . nothing. It's so frustrating! I seem to last too long and then, when I can't come, I finally lose my erection. Sometimes I've sort of faked it and told my partner that I've had a dry orgasm or I just stop and say that I'm too tired. I know she's confused about this, but I can't seem to talk to her about it. I'm fifty-one and have been drinking more heavily than usual recently. I'm also very tense about things at work. But when I lose my erection, we just stop all touching. We roll away from each other, nothing's said, and I know my partner isn't usually sexually satisfied either.

You're describing delayed ejaculation, which is sometimes found in men over the age of fifty. There are many possible causes of delayed ejaculation (you can read more on this disorder in appendix A) such as depression, medication side effects, fatigue, anxiety, excessive masturbation, alcohol or drug abuse, sex that has become too routine, and the discomfort requesting additional or specific stimulation.

You mention your increase in alcohol consumption, and you really need to look at this, as it may be contributing to the inhibited ejaculation. Your work stress may also be a cause, as you're probably distracted and anxious because of it. Additionally, it's important to transition to intercourse only when your sexual arousal is very high, not just at the onset of an erection. Experiment with different types of stimulation.

During masturbation, pay attention to possible orgasm triggers, such as different positions, types of movement, speed, and pelvic muscle tension. Your masturbation technique may not be something you can easily use during partner sex. There's a sexercise at the end of this chapter that can guide you in exploring this issue. Remember to talk with your partner about what kinds of stimulation, verbal expression, and stroking you need.

Be sure to talk to your partner about the stress at work and your increased alcohol consumption. Let her know what you're learning about your sexual arousal. You'll need to reassure her that the ejaculatory difficulty isn't her fault. Your partner can be your ally in this journey as you explore possible causes and solutions. Be sure to use other sexual techniques and sensual interaction when intercourse or orgasm isn't satisfying. You and your partner will benefit from all types of playful, erotic, and caressing activity. Try some VENIS.

❧❧❧

Beyond Intercourse   There are many ways to feel turned on and satisfied without having penis-in-the-vagina sex.

- Sometimes referred to as outercourse, rubbing the penis between the breasts or thighs or buttocks can add variety. This is especially nice for couples who are dealing with vaginal pain issues.
- The "summer of '69" takes on new meaning . . . that position can be a turn-on for some.
- Oral stimulation for males or females is sometimes a great appetizer, or it may be the entrée.
- Anal stimulation is also fun for some.
- Hitting those hot spots with a vibrator can create quite a buzz.
- Mutual masturbation is very erotic.
- Rubbing or manual stimulation is a great use of friction.

Good Sex Should Be Mind-Blowing Every Time

Was it good for you . . . did you come . . . was that as great as last time . . . am I your best lover? These are some loaded questions! Wow, there can be a lot of pressure involved in this intimate act—sex—which is meant to bring a great deal of pleasure! Sometimes it may feel like you're preparing for an exam or have just completed a rigorous competition! Who wants that? However, it seems that we have a lot riding on the notion that really hot, erotic, earthmoving sex should be the goal for every sexual encounter. Everyone would like that, but is it reasonable and possible?

There are many books available that encourage or teach couples how to increase eroticism and passion. And this is certainly a worthy pursuit. But what about the occasions when there's just too much stress in the day, or getting to orgasm seems like climbing the tallest mountain, or the erectile medication didn't work very well?

Dr. Metz and Dr. McCarthy have written about the concept of "good-enough sex."[3] This model encourages couples to view sexuality as a lifelong process involving changes from young adulthood to older age. The good-enough sex model accepts that every sexual encounter isn't perfect and that the quality of sex varies for each experience. Metz and McCarthy urge healthy couples to adopt the notion that sex is "very good" about 20–25 percent of the time; "good" about 40–60 percent of the time; "fair" but unremarkable 15–20 percent of the time; and dissatisfying or dysfunctional 5–15 percent of the time.

In therapy, Lance and Laura spoke about ongoing sexual problems. Laura had difficulty becoming aroused and found that she usually only had an orgasm when she was very rested and Lance gave her oral sex. She was disappointed that the simple act of intercourse alone didn't lead to an easy orgasm for her.

Additionally, Lance was discovering that, at times, he was experiencing rapid ejaculation. This didn't occur each time they had sex, but he found that it was more likely when he was fatigued and when sex became infrequent.

Their therapist talked to Lance and Laura about the good-enough sex model and explained that they were within the normal range for healthy couples. Discovering that their sexual interaction fit the model helped Laura and Lance accept that there was nothing abnormal about their sexual relationship. They also learned, from examining their patterns and sexual needs, more about what they required in order for sex to be optimal. They decided that they would each make a list of what they needed and wanted: emotionally, environmentally, physically, sensually, and erotically. Lance and Laura sat down and read over their lists and discussed what was shared and what was new information. Here are their lists:

Laura: I need to feel rested and relaxed. I'd like the house to be fairly picked up (not too messy). I love the backrubs you give and that always helps me relax. I'd like to try reading or watching something erotic together. And you know that I love it when you talk dirty and also when you give me oral sex. When sex is a little disappointing for us, I'd like it if we could just cuddle afterward and not move away from each other right away.

Lance: It seems that I need to either not wait too many days between times we have sex or I need to go ahead and masturbate a little more often (if you aren't in the mood, Laura). I need to watch how much sleep I'm getting and also how much I'm exercising. I love giving and receiving oral sex and would like more of that. I'd also like to try some new positions.

This shared information gave Lance and Laura a lot to talk about regarding what they each felt they needed and what new interaction they'd like to try. They discussed how they would like to handle the situation when either one or both were sexually dissatisfied. They determined that they would enjoy cuddling and giving sensual massages. Additionally, Lance and Laura talked about being open to trying again on another day, without too much time passing, and that they would understand that this wasn't rejection, just a date for another time.

Orgasms Should Come Easily If You Know What to Do

The ability to orgasm during sex may be achieved rather easily for some people. When hormones are at adequate levels, sexual technique is effective, the relationship is new, and there's still much to be discovered about each other, sexual satisfaction is usually high. However, males and females are more likely to orgasm with more consistency during masturbation than during partner sex. In fact, 75 percent of men, but only 29 percent of women, always have an orgasm during sex with their partner.[4] In contrast, about 80 percent of men, compared to 60 percent of women, report that they usually or always have an orgasm when masturbating.

There are many possible reasons for orgasm inconsistency within the genders. Whether with masturbation or intercourse, males and females are not all the same when it comes to sexual arousal and ease of orgasm. At times, achieving orgasm may be very reliable and dependable, but many things can interfere with orgasm. Some of these are changes in hormone levels, issues around sexual technique, fatigue, medication, interpersonal conflicts, stress, substance overuse—the list is endless.

Arousal techniques and positions that are used in masturbation, for males and females, may not transfer well to partner sex. A woman who consistently uses her vibrator or an idiosyncratic style during self-stimulation may find that her technique doesn't translate with ease to sex with her partner. A male may prefer a personal technique that doesn't work well with a partner, such as the use of porn. You'll find some tips for transitioning from self-stimulation to partner interaction in the sexercises portion of this chapter.

Sex Should Be Spontaneous

Madeline spoke in therapy about the change in her relationship with her partner. She recalled that, when they were first together, they would often call one another at work and agree to meet for lunch in a nearby park. Once there, they would usually find themselves making out to the point of orgasm for one or both. This midday interaction seemed to fuel Madeline and her partner to be sexual again in the afternoon or evening after work. She explained, "I miss our spontaneous rendezvous in the park. Sometimes I would even take off my bra or panties before we met and it was so exciting to see his surprise and enjoyment! He'd also surprise me with spontaneous picnics in our living room and that would lead to sex on the floor. What has happened to us? Now we just go through the motions of our days; we meet at home after work and sometimes we make love at night, but it's so routine!"

But was it ever really *that* spontaneous? Even when dating, most of us plan what we'll wear, rehearse what we might say during a date, determine what perfume or cologne to use, and give a lot of thought to which restaurant might have the most romantic atmosphere. It takes planning! However, when the relationship has lingered, the passion and spontaneity may have languished.

Leaving the romance up to chance is risky—and we're not talking about the fun, exciting kind of risk! Without planning and intentionality, sexual fires usually dim. Planned spontaneity can include all sorts of sexy and fun interactions. It's intriguing to plan a surprising rendezvous or outing with the purpose of keeping the love alive or the sex hot.

"Planned Spontaneity" for Great Dates
- Go for a picnic
- Make out in the car
- Take a cooking class

- Go dancing
- Go canoeing
- Sip wine on the back porch
- Eat fondue together in the nude
- Take salsa lessons
- Go for a bike trip
- Visit wine country
- Hike in the woods
- Have a couple's massage
- Take a couple's Tantra workshop

COMMON MISTAKEN ASSUMPTIONS

Fantasies Are Dangerous

Many people use fantasy during masturbation and while engaged in partner sex. The themes of sexual fantasies vary and may include images that are unusual or even unacceptable in our culture. However, most sexual fantasies are simply the expression of sensuous longings and free us from societal constraints. The great majority of fantasies don't indicate that we desire the behaviors or the person or persons in the erotic images. They are simply a means by which we can heighten our erotic focus and arousal.

Can sexual fantasies be shared with your partner? Sometimes private images may be best kept private, but good communication about sharing fantasies can help a couple decide what's off limits. Fantasies can have a variety of functions, including enhancement of self-esteem and attractiveness, increasing sexual arousal, rehearsal of future sexual possibilities, satisfying curiosity, preserving a pleasant memory, and facilitating orgasm.[5] Please refer to the resources section to find books regarding fantasy.

SEXUAL HEALING

I'm in a gay relationship, and my partner and I talked the other day about possibly sharing our fantasies with each other. We were both a little hesitant. Is it a good idea?

Good question! Sexual fantasies, as noted above, have many positive functions. Sharing these fantasies with a lover can be a bit tricky. Verbalizing the fantasy may increase or enhance arousal and that would be great; however, some partners may hear the fantasy and feel jealousy, insecurity, or even disgust. Maltz and Boss suggest two guidelines for sharing: (1) share in safety and in steps; you can always stop if you feel judged or misunderstood, and (2) select what to share; you may not want to give all the details.[6] If you and your partner decide to enact a fantasy, be sure that you talk about ground rules beforehand. Sometimes acting out fantasies can threaten the relationship, lower self-esteem, interfere with intimacy, or become risky. Talk about stopping if the interaction becomes awkward or threatening. However, acting out fantasies can also bring spice and intrigue. So be sure to talk this issue over with your partner.

Low Desire Means You Need Testosterone

The debate over the use of testosterone has been going on for some time now. When males complain of low desire, one of the first steps in treatment is to evaluate testosterone levels. Many times, the augmentation of testosterone will prove to be helpful for a man with diminished libido. However, even for men, the use of testosterone will not always alleviate the desire dilemma. There may be other reasons, besides low testosterone, for low desire, such as relationship conflict, overuse of or dependency on porn, a variant arousal pattern (such as a fetish), or an unsatisfactory treatment for an erectile issue.

Pharmaceutical companies are attempting to find a treatment for females with low desire. Some women are given off-label prescriptions for testosterone; however, there are dangers in using testosterone, such as negative interactions with other medications, possible side effects, and unforeseen long-term consequences for women's health. Use of drugs to treat low libido may obscure the wide range of diversity and variability among females regarding normal healthy sexual functioning.

The hormonal issues involved in low desire for females may account for only a small percentage of female sexual problems. In a 2008 study, Leanne Nicholls, PsyD, used a survey to determine how 49 women viewed their sexual difficulties.[7] Sixty-five percent attributed their sexual problems to relationship issues, 20 percent to contextual factors, and 8 percent to psychological issues. Only 7 percent cited medical problems as the cause of their sexual distress. Therefore, it's very important to explore all possible causes of low libido in females, looking at the biological, psychological, and relational contributors to desire.

If You Don't Orgasm, There's Something Wrong

For both men and women, there's a lot of pressure to orgasm during sex. It's a great idea, but it is not always achievable or even desirable! Men often equate good sex with their own orgasm and that of their partner. Women often feel that they *must* orgasm and that their sexual task is to bring their partner to a mind-blowing climax. Orgasm is certainly a worthy goal, but what happens when IT just doesn't happen?

For males, not having an orgasm with intercourse can be met with anything from disappointment to sheer panic. As we have discussed, many things can interfere with desire, arousal, and orgasm. We need to accept that not every sexual encounter ends in orgasm. If we turn to other erotic or sensual scenarios when orgasm eludes us, then the sexual and emotional relationship doesn't have to suffer.

For many females, orgasm is difficult to achieve during partner sex. This might be due to many of the same issues that plague men and their orgasms—hormones, lowered desire, illness, medication, and relationship conflict. Females have the added challenge that clitoral stimulation is important but not always easily realized. The pressure to reach orgasm may be extremely detrimental to female desire and arousal. It's not a good idea to have to perform for a partner. This may lead to the age-old issue of "whether to fake it or not." It's better to address the challenge of orgasm openly and honestly. Not all women desire orgasm with every encounter and many feel very satisfied with the sexual experience, even without the Big Bang.

Low Desire Means Something's Wrong in the Relationship

It *is* true that a lack of desire may indicate that there is something askew in the relationship, but this also can be a false and misleading assumption. We may feel fearful that our low desire is rooted in our relationship problems or in a loss of *being in love*. But remember—initial attraction and excitement will wane over time. The hormones and neurotransmitters that once ignited flames of passion will eventually diminish. We will then find that our once-erotic relationship has dimmed to only small embers with barely discernible heat. This can be confusing as we might begin to wonder if our loss of sexual intensity is ushering in a loss of love.

Some of us are able to partner effortlessly in many areas of our relationship. Perhaps we're able to parent easily, manage money simply, and find equanimity in household duties, but we still tiptoe around the area of eroticism and passion. Why is this? We might have inadequate sexual knowledge, difficulty discussing sexual needs or concerns, shame surrounding our body or sexual urges, fear of intimacy, or the inability to share our internal erotic world. For some, it may be very difficult to be an erotic person within a long-term relationship or to be sexually uninhibited with each other. This can be challenging, and there's more on this in chapter 9.

Fix the Relationship and Desire Will Increase

This assumption is related to the previous one, that a low libido indicates there's something amiss in the relationship. When we assume that the relationship distance or conflict is contributing to low desire, we may attempt to spend more time together, share intimate details of our lives, and connect about the kids and work. Undoubtedly, if there is a great deal of arguing and conflict, learning how to communicate respectfully and effectively will help us feel more positively toward one another. It's not uncommon for women to report that they need more closeness and intimacy in order to feel sexually safe and open.

Unfortunately, clearing the air, learning to fight fairly, and becoming closer friends does not always translate into increased passion. No doubt, it's a great step in the right direction! Without kindness, respect, and connection, sexual desire will likely not last long, but getting along doesn't necessarily guarantee hot sex.

So, what do couples need to do in order to generate erotic desire? Answering this question is complex and every couple will need to explore their own paths to passion. A good place to start is in thinking about how to anticipate and long for sexual activity. We've included much more on this topic in chapter 9.

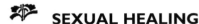 SEXUAL HEALING

My partner and I are such good friends. We've been together for three years now and I love coming home to her. We have a great deck and sit out on it most evenings, just talking, sharing about the day, and laughing about crazy stuff. I love that, and I love her! But the problem is that I feel like we're both getting a bit bored in the bedroom. I know that I am. I'd like to try some new things. Maybe some toys or new positions. I don't know how to bring it up though. I don't want her to feel that I'm dissatisfied or that she's not turning me on. She does turn me on, but I'd really like to take it up a notch. What do I do?

We think that's a great place to start in your conversation with your partner—assure her that you are very turned on by her, enjoy the sex you have, and really love her. This is an example of a relationship that's working in many areas—intimacy, connection, fun—but that doesn't inoculate you against the sexual monotony that sometimes ensues when the relationship is long-term. You can suggest that there is something that you've either read about recently, seen in a film, or heard someone talking about and that you've always wanted to try it. Just throw it out there, but be open to her ideas and to the fact that she might not be as interested in the same activities. Ask her if there are things that she's been wanting to try, but has felt awkward about asking. You could try writing some of your ideas down and then sharing them. Enjoy the exploration. You've got such a great foundation for this type of communication!

Everyone's Having Great Sex, Except Us

The media has contributed to the idea that everyone is having great hot sex. Celebrities talk openly about their sexual experiences; videos surface showing couples in erotic interactions; and every women's magazine has an article about new positions and techniques to try! Are we suffering then from a new phenomenon of *sexual comparison anxiety* created by our culture?

Comparison to others usually takes us down an unsatisfying path, whether it has to do with sexual expectations, wealth, children's achievements, or physical appearance. It may be surprising, but reassuring, to know that at some point in about 50 percent of marriages, couples experience inhibited desire or a desire discrepancy. As defined by McCarthy and McCarthy, approximately one in five married couples has a no-sex marriage (sex occurring less than ten times a year).[8] Additionally, the authors point out that about 15 percent of married couples have a low-sex marriage (sex occurring less than twenty-five times a year or less than every other week). Even one in three cohabitating couples who have been together more than two years have a no-sex relationship.

Whether the comparison has to do with sexual frequency or sexual satisfaction or experimentation, it's critical that couples take a problem-solving approach to this issue. Discuss perceptions regarding sexual experiences and beliefs about these expectations. Examine fears and anxieties, the pressures to fit some stereotyped ideal of sexual fulfillment, and your own unique sexual pattern. It's self-defeating to compare your sexual relationship to what may or may not be the reality of others.

This Is Just a Phase; Sex Will Improve

Paul brought up in therapy that, among other issues, he felt that his sex life with his partner, Patty, had diminished to possibly once a month or less. He and Patty argued for a bit about how long it had been since they'd had sex and what the causes were for their infrequency. Finally, they both agreed that sex had been put on the back burner due to stresses in the family: a teenager with drug issues, Patty's ill mother, and the strain of Paul's loss of income in his real estate business. Both of them agreed that they had hoped that things would return to normal (sex about once a week, usually weekend mornings), but neither of them had talked about their concerns until now. The tension had built as they felt more distant and less satisfied sexually and emotionally.

Often couples allow distance to develop, while hoping that somehow the detachment will eventually lessen and the relationship will return to its previous intimacy. Perhaps the warmth and sexual energy is restored for some lucky couples without much conscious effort. However, most of us find that time passes and there's still no resolution to the distance.

Without attacking the other's lack of sexual desire or availability, we need to discuss reclaiming the sexual relationship. We need to carve

out time for reconnecting with each other and each person will need
to dedicate time to his or her own individual sensual exploration. There
are often many concerns that take the focus and energy away from the
couple and even away from an individual's own sexual awareness. A
great place to start is with a discussion about how to support one another
so that the distractions of daily life are not overwhelming. It's then important for each person to set aside time to tune into the other, sensually
and erotically. If there's still a lot of resistance or conflict around finding
time for sex, it might be necessary to talk with a relationship therapist or
sex therapist to determine if there are serious couple dynamics or sexual
concerns interfering.

   ## SEXUAL HEALING

I feel guilty, but I feel like our sex has become really boring. I think it's
been about two months since my partner and I had sex, and this is becoming a pattern for us. We've lived together for about five years, and
I don't want to lose this relationship. But I just avoid him at night and
I know that I'm just hoping that things will get better in time. I do this
with a lot of things in my life: I put off my papers in graduate school
until the last minute, I don't bring up issues with friends when I should,
and now this. I'm a big chicken! I just don't want to talk about it; I guess
I'm scared because I don't know what we'll be able to do about it.

*This is a really honest assessment of yourself! You seem to see a pattern
in your approach to life, in general. Perhaps you've learned that this
works for you in some way. But probably you'll find that in many issues
in your life, leaving things to "fix themselves," so to speak, isn't usually
the wisest method. When it comes to sex, it's not a tactic that we would
recommend. Can you remember all the reasons that sex was good for
you two in the past? Think about what you did at the beginning of the
relationship that made sex really hot. Chapter 9 has some ideas about
how to spice things up, such as using fantasy and toys. You might bring
this up to your partner by saying, "I feel worried that we're getting into
a rut sexually. I have been reading about some new sexual techniques
and positions that I'd like to try. What do you think?" Reading this book*

together will give you both some more ideas about what to try and how to talk about sex.

MOVING ACROSS THE BRIDGE

It's natural for all of us to fall into the trap of making assumptions about what sex *should* be like. Often these beliefs are self-limiting and can lead to expectations that are unrealistic or even harmful to emotional or sexual intimacy.

How do you resolve the misguided beliefs? Sometimes the answer to the mistaken perception can be found in educating yourself about these opinions or expectations, such as reading this book and others in our resources section. Other times, it's necessary to sit down together and discuss the assumptions that the two of you have. The dialogue can then allow you to voice anxieties and express the faulty demands that you may have been placing on yourself or on one another. Freeing yourselves from these lofty expectations releases you to enjoy your sexual relationship and grow together as lovers.

SEXERCISES

I. Consider what you would like to have, given the best of all worlds, when pursuing a sexual relationship with your partner. Using your journal, write about what you'd like to have in each of the following areas in order to feel at your best sexually. Remember that you can explore sensual massage or other types of pleasuring without going to intercourse or orgasm each time.

- What would I like the *environment* to be (in the bedroom, someplace else in the house, in a hotel room, someplace I've never tried, etc.)?
- How would I like to feel *physically* (for example, some people dislike having sex after a big meal or when they have a headache)?

- What would I like to be feeling *emotionally* in our relationship (for instance, some individuals want to feel especially close, while others don't require that)?
- What special *sensual extras* would I like to have present (candles, music, lighting, fireplace, hot tub, food, wine, dancing, etc.)?
- What specific *kinds of touch* would I like to have (where exactly would I like to be touched, what sort of touch turns me on the most)?
- What would I like to try that might *increase eroticism* (toys, more or less verbal talk, new positions, erotica, etc.)?

After writing down your desires in each of these areas, take some time to talk to your partner about what you would like to try to incorporate into your sexual style.

II. Consider the good-enough sex model explained earlier in this chapter: sex is "very good" about 20–25 percent of the time; "good" about 40–60 percent of the time; "fair" but unremarkable 15–20 percent of the time; and dissatisfying or dysfunctional 5–15 percent of the time.

Think about your own sexual expectations and the pressures you may be feeling about your performance or outcome. Write about this and then talk with your partner about how these unrealistic expectations have been affecting you both.

III. If you have found that orgasms are much more predictable and more easily attained when self-stimulating than with partner sex, consider practicing ways to transfer this method to partner sex. You'll need to set aside about a half hour or more. Make sure that you're relaxed and won't be disturbed by anyone. Set the stage as much as possible to enhance your erotic senses. Begin stimulating yourself in your usual manner, paying attention to your body's position and your technique. Consider whether your style is similar to sexual positions and methods of arousal that you and your partner use.

In order to make the transition from masturbation to partner sex more fulfilling, it's best if you can take what you're learning about your personal arousal style and merge it with partner sex. It may be necessary to try stimulating yourself with the hand that you don't usually use for masturbation so that your sexual response is not as predictable. You might start in your favorite position for self-stimulation and then move into a position that you would more likely use with your partner. When thinking about what you commonly do during intercourse, imagine what it would be like to use similar speed, pressure, techniques, fantasy, and movements that you employ in masturbation. As a female, if you normally use a vibrator, you can practice using it initially for stimulation and then attempt to continue stimulation manually. Of course, mutual masturbation can be a real turn-on for many couples. Additionally, reaching orgasm before, during, or after actual intercourse is very acceptable and healthy.

IV. Take each of the assumptions explained in the book and consider whether you and your partner have fallen into its trap. Talk about each one of the seven beliefs and its effect on your sexual relationship:

1. Fantasies are dangerous.
2. Low desire means you need testosterone.
3. If you don't orgasm, there's something wrong.
4. Low desire means something's wrong in the relationship.
5. Fix the relationship and desire will increase.
6. Everyone's having great sex, except us.
7. This is just a phase; sex will improve.

V. The expectation that sex always equals intercourse can be damaging for couples because it leads to performance anxiety and doesn't transfer well for couples as they age or have illness. Take some time, using your imagination, and create scenes in which you and your partner increase eroticism but don't include intercourse. Think about locations, in the bedroom and otherwise, where you might enjoy sensual massage. Consider types of touch that would exclude genitals, but still be very erotic. Remember the make-out sessions that you used to have, perhaps as a teenager, and imagine doing that with your partner, clothed or partially clothed. Consider all the means by which you might arouse each other—manually, orally, by rubbing, or with toys. Now take these images and talk with your partner, whisper them in his or her ear, or write them down and share them.

8

INTERPRETATIONS OF THE RELATIONSHIP DANCE

Negotiating the Steps

I had an affair, and my partner says that he's forgiven me. But I feel that the affair is still haunting us. I don't think I've even forgiven myself.

—Female, age 41

- Do you and your partner argue about who's right?
- Do you avoid your partner sexually when you're angry?
- Are you holding onto resentment from your partner's affair?
- Do you find yourself spending hours looking at porn?
- Do you withhold sex?

"Why didn't someone tell me that being in a long-term relationship was going to be so rough?" "If I had known then what I know now, I wouldn't have gotten involved with the guy!" We hear these exclamations so often! A friend of ours, after four marriages, wisely puts it this way, "Ah, marriage . . . it's not for the faint of heart!" No long-term relationship, whether it is a marriage or not, is easy.

Imagine the relationship as a dance. Sometimes the dance partners are very close, holding each other chest-to-chest, hips swaying, and eyes locked on each other. At other times, the dance partners step away from one another and momentarily lose contact. When the partners are in harmony, the dance is graceful and well choreographed. But we've all seen dancers who are awkward and even dangerously uncoordinated. Toes are stepped on and arguments ensue over who's going to lead.

It's challenging to learn the steps in the relationship dance! Some of us have had masterful dance instructors and the opportunity to polish our movements, leading to comfortable, easy interaction. Others are natural dancers with innate agility and grace. Still others of us have never quite learned the steps and we seem clumsy as we move across the floor in this relationship dance.

Let's look at movements in this dance of intimacy that may have led many of us to think about walking off the dance floor for good! When a relationship has become strained, emotional closeness and sex will often be put on the back burner. We'll examine the following relationship challenges: avoidance of sex, power struggles, conflict, affairs, and pornography use.

NO THANKS, I'LL SIT THIS ONE OUT!

Dan and Denise, a couple who had been together for about twenty years, came to therapy because sex had diminished to about once every three or four months. When talking about this issue, Denise and Dan both agreed there was little affection or touching outside of the bedroom. Denise avoided Dan physically because she had recently found that her orgasm was almost nonexistent due to perimenopause. Dan knew very little about Denise's problems with orgasm and avoided her physically due to his fear of rejection. Dan also explained that he was confused about how to show Denise affection and love without Denise feeling pressured to have sex. Dan and Denise agreed that they both felt awkward even thinking about engaging in sex when they felt almost like complete strangers to each other. Their therapist helped the couple talk specifically about what each needed and wanted regarding touch and connection. Specifically, Denise needed time to explore her orgasm, both by herself and with Dan.

Does this sound familiar . . . a relationship in which avoidance and silence have become the norm? At times, we avoid difficulty by taking an exit ramp in a relationship. What are exit ramps? They're all the things that take us off the road leading to a deeper and more fulfilling relationship with our partner. Exit ramps might be working too many hours, watching TV instead of talking, playing computer games, drinking, having an affair, being overly involved with your kids' lives, even exercising! There are a lot of possible exits!

Exits may allow us to avoid sex with our partners. The following questions can shed light on the causes of avoidance:

Why do I avoid my partner?

- Do I feel angry?
- Do I feel misunderstood?
- Do I feel unappreciated?
- Am I just too tired to care?
- Do I feel I'm not being heard?
- Do I think that my partner just wants sex, but isn't interested in me as a person?
- Am I embarrassed about my body or about some sexual act that I think my partner may want to do?
- Do I feel anxious about my sexual performance?

�֎ SEXUAL HEALING

I've avoided my partner for so long now; I don't even know how to begin to reconnect. But I'm beginning to feel like I miss my partner and want to start having sex again. We rarely touch, and I can't even imagine how to approach him. Can you help?

It becomes awkward to start touching again in a sexual manner when too much time has passed between affectionate and playful interaction. It's best not to let more than a week or two go by without some kind of reconnection in a sexual or sensual way. It may not be that you have sex every week or two, but it's important to have time together that's focused on rekindling affection and emotional ties. Go ahead and talk to your partner about how awkward it feels now that you've slipped away from one another. Put your heads together to come up with some creative means by which to start affectionate and sexy touching again. Think of ways to incorporate couple fun into your life.

✻ ✻ ✻

"I feel like we've become roommates." One of the most common reasons for avoidance of sex is the issue of feeling disconnected. It's challenging to go from talking about the kids' schedules, the bills that need to be paid, and why his mother keeps calling, to hot and heavy action under the covers! When you're taking care of everyday issues in life and get into routines, it begins to be awkward to look at our partner in a sexual way. Fatigue, spats, and familiarity throw cold water on the heat of passion. We all remember the beginning of the relationship—you can't wait to see each other, you think her laugh is cute, and he tells such fascinating stories! After a few months or a few years, you begin to dread the sound of his car coming in the drive, her laugh grates on your very last nerve, and his stories are so boring—you've heard them all before!

When there's a feeling of distance and disconnection, it's important to look for ways to bring some "play" back into the relationship. But how can we rekindle passion in a relationship when it's fallen into the same old dull routine? A weekly date night needs to be on the calendar and can consist of simply going for a walk or a more elegant date of dinner and dancing. Some couples enjoy meeting at a bar and pretending that they've just met for the first time, then indulging in a sexy conversation about what each would enjoy in bed! Going away for a night—no kids, no TV, no phone—can rekindle desire that may have seemed a distant memory. Plan an evening to massage each other or relax together in a hot tub. Go for a bike ride and enjoy wine outdoors. It's fun to use your imagination, talk to your partner about things that were exciting while dating, and relive a memory. If we leave the playfulness up to chance, thinking that it's not romantic to plan or that it will "just happen," it more than likely won't. And certainly nothing sexy will happen!

WILL YOU *PLEASE* LET ME LEAD?

Who's in charge here, anyway? Who gets to be right? The issue of power struggles in relationships probably dates back to the beginning of time. We can hear it now, "I've been waiting for hours for you to come home! I've told you a thousand times that I don't like it when you hunt and gather for days on end! Wash your own loin cloth and fix your own boar stew!"

In therapy, we hear the age-old debate of who's right and who's wrong. She likes dinner at a certain time; her partner needs to work late. He wants to buy a new big-screen TV; his partner feels that they need money for the kids' activities. She likes to snuggle after dinner; he thinks snuggling should definitely lead to some under-the-shirt action. Shall we take a vote? Inevitably, there's no clear winner in these situations. When the power struggles are many and ongoing, couples usually pull away from one another and build a protective wall of anger or avoidance. Couples often express a feeling of disappointment regarding the power struggles they encounter in long-term relationships. The loss of "it's us against the world" is distressing to couples. Instead of feeling close and protected by their partners, people within contentious relationships express feelings of isolation and betrayal.

Gottman and Gottman, research psychologists, suggest that many couples can make peace with their differences when they look for the "longing" in the complaints being uttered.[1] Asking ourselves about the "longing" in our partner's complaint can shed light on what it is that he or she would like or desires. When a partner complains about too much TV watching, it might be accurate to look at the complaint as actually a desire for time to spend together and enhance connectedness.

It's helpful to also explore our own common complaints to see what the underlying desire might be. For instance, a person who longs for physical closeness in order to feel connected and supported may, instead of expressing his desire for closeness, actually complain or criticize his partner for lack of sex, low desire, or for any number of things that take the partner's time. Rather than stating, "You never seem to want sex any more. What's wrong with you?" the expression of longing opens up the dialogue ("I miss our closeness and the fun sex we used to have. I love to touch your body and it feels so good to make out.").

SEXUAL HEALING

I really want my partner to try different sexual positions, but she's very reluctant to do much more than the missionary position. I have shown her articles that indicate that people are much more experimental than we are, but she just makes excuses for not trying stuff. Don't you think I'm right about this? We need some variety!

Talk with your partner about whether she has fears about being experimental. Perhaps there are body image issues that she's struggling with and she may be uncomfortable exposing her body in sexual positions other than the missionary position. Additionally, she might feel that if she agrees to try another position, you'll want that position all the time, and it might not be "her thing." Or she may fear that you will keep pushing the envelope to try something new with each sexual encounter and she may not be ready for that or ever want that.

This is one of those dilemmas that can cause an impasse which may never actually be solved. There's a myth that, if we just talk things out enough and hammer away at our own brilliant point, we'll eventually convince the other person of our opinion. Research has indicated that this is not true. Some problems in relationships are solvable, others are modifiable, and still others remain unsolvable. Talk to your partner about whether your differences in this area really have no resolution. It will take a great deal of patience and tolerance to come to terms with this, but it may be necessary that you develop an acceptance of your differences. You may have to agree to disagree!

IF YOU STEP ON MY TOES ONE MORE TIME, I'M OUTTA HERE!

Ouch! Relationships can be a pain! It hurts to be ignored, put down, or criticized. When we've been hurt time after time, we may want to get the heck outta there! Many once-loving couples slip into constant bickering or stop almost all dialogue because of arguing. When the relationship is filled with a great deal of tension, there isn't much room for sexual fun.

Relationship conflict, stored anger, and sexual problems are like a tangled ball of threads, with no clear beginning or ending. There seems to be no obvious place to start the process of healing because one issue often leads to another and then back again to the original problem or even a new one. It's difficult to separate the threads and thoroughly deal with the sexual ones, while keeping all the relational threads in a neat pile someplace else. We really have to address both the sexual and the relationship issues simultaneously.

We believe it's best to keep the anger issues outside of the bedroom, while restoring intimacy and trust in the bedroom. This can be challenging! When a couple has conflict, anger, or resentment smoldering in their relationship, it's advisable to talk about these issues in a neutral environment. The kitchen table when both are rested and the kids are at the neighbor's may be a safe and calm setting. Sessions with a therapist can help clarify the problems and shed light on possible solutions. Discussing difficult matters can even be handled at a restaurant, at times, with both partners agreeing to keep it civil. It's ill-advised to come to bed with an agenda of resentments that need to be discussed right then and there. Couples need to keep the bedroom for sleeping, touching, caressing, and the erotic. You may need to go back to the tips for communicating about difficult topics in chapter 6.

🌿 SEXUAL HEALING

I love my partner and we usually have great sex, but we argue a lot. It seems like we keep rehashing the same old stuff. If we've been arguing and he comes to bed and puts the moves on me, it just pisses me off! How could he think I'm in the mood when we just finished yelling at each other?

We hear this so often in therapy! Men and women appear to want the same thing—intimacy and connection—but we go about it in very different ways. Men usually feel emotionally close when they have sex, but women often need the emotional connection before they have sex. Never agree to unwanted sex. Coercive sex is never okay! It's important to let your partner know that you want to have sex at some point, but that you aren't in the mood right after an argument. Take a break from the tension after you've been arguing. You don't have to solve all arguments in one sitting. And some arguments will never be solved, quite frankly! Find ways to open a window to each other again.

🌿 🌿 🌿

Tips for Dealing with Conflict:
- Remember that disagreements can illuminate issues that the two of you need to understand.
- Don't argue the point of "right vs. wrong," as this can be an endless and frustrating discussion. Acknowledge differences and try to accept your partner's style and approach to life.

- Keep your anger response/behavior at a low to moderate level. Don't sink to defensiveness, criticism, blaming, name-calling, threats, or physical violence.
- If you find that one or both of you is building a wall without an avenue to open dialogue, find a time to sit with each other and explore what's taking place in your negotiation style.
- Approach your partner's feelings and statements with the notion that there is a logical and legitimate reason for them. Ask open-ended questions to seek understanding, "Tell me about . . ." or "What do you think you need at this point in order to . . . ?"
- Share responsibility for problems in the relationship.
- Focus on one problem at a time and try to stay in the present.
- Discuss problematic behaviors and actions; don't attack character.
- Acknowledge the emotions behind what each of you are saying when discussing something of importance.
- Express appreciation for mature and productive conversations.
- If your conflict is leading to distance in your sexual relationship, address this as a desire and longing, rather than a criticism or threat.
- If you find that you can't explore your differences productively, find help from a therapist.

"CAN I CUT IN?"

The relationship dance is traditionally choreographed for two partners. For most couples, there really isn't room for a third, particularly when it involves the secrecy of an affair. When a third party enters the picture, the status quo is altered and an imbalance takes place, even if the affair has not been revealed.

Is an affair always about sex? No. Some affairs are emotional relationships and there's little physical contact. Other affairs are almost exclusively sexual in nature. And still others have the components of both emotional and sexual involvement. Emotional affairs can be as damaging and threatening to a relationship as sexual affairs.

Is an affair always about wanting to leave the relationship? It depends. Sometimes infidelity is the result of acting on an impulse in a situation in which there is the belief that the sexual encounter is unlikely to be revealed. Other times, an affair is a means, either consciously or unconsciously, to explore options and make comparisons. At times, the affair is an "exit affair" in which a person seeks out an involvement, perhaps hoping that the new relationship will ease her pain or loneliness and help her to leave the present troubled relationship.

Does an affair mean that the primary relationship is a flawed one and that the love between the original two has withered? Again, not necessarily. At times, a person finds herself shutting out her partner or feeling shut out by her partner. She and her partner may simply have little time to devote to each other, and she might seek someone with whom she can talk. She probably didn't set out to destroy her primary relationship or to create a new one, but she finds herself with a fresh and exciting emotional connection. Once the affair has begun, she then feels that her primary relationship must be, in some way, flawed and she begins to justify the other relationship.

Reasons for affairs are many. Couples drift apart, conflicts poison the relationship, work takes the partners away from each other, sexual disorders result in frustration and the search for something different. And the list goes on. Many couples find themselves building barriers between each other, sometimes even innocently, while opening doors to others.

Jill came to therapy to explore and heal from her own infidelity. She expressed that she felt very frustrated at home. She and her partner, Jim, seemed to spend little time together. Jim rarely helped around the house, he had recently spent a huge amount of money on a golf weekend with his college friends, and Jill felt that he didn't listen to her when she talked about work. At the office, Jill had found herself opening up to Craig, her coworker. Craig seemed kind, talked openly with her about his past, and didn't even play golf! Jill had slowly opened the door to an intimate relationship with Craig. She explained that she was almost unaware of how easily she fell into the intimate sexual relationship with Craig.

Infidelity is a challenging and complex wound from which to heal. Affairs cost both partners and the relationship a great deal in terms of commitment and trust. If a person chooses to stay with their partner, healing *can* follow infidelity. Part of the healing process involves understanding the meaning of the affair to both parties and committing to the renewal of trust in the relationship. As with any wound, some injuries from affairs may run very deep, and it will take extraordinary measures to restore the relationship to health. When the affair is discovered or revealed, the couple will need to know how to mend the abrasions in the relationship. Without effective communication, the couple may "pick at the wound" and healing can be impossible. The injury needs to be thoroughly cleaned and treated; simply bandaging the wound won't do.

When the discovery of an affair is made, a rollercoaster ride of emotions follows. It's challenging to talk about what has happened without falling into arguments and accusations. Couples need to take time to heal from the affair and seek help as options are considered. Each situation is unique and there are inevitably underlying issues to consider that may have been festering unnoticed or ignored in the background of the relationship.

 ## SEXUAL HEALING

I had an affair and I have confessed to my partner that I'm still in contact with the person I had the affair with. I run into her at work and I continue to take her phone calls. I want to stay with my current partner and make my relationship work, but I seem drawn back to the other woman.

It's impossible to do any real work toward rebuilding your relationship as long as the affair partner remains in the picture. Secrecy between you and the other woman will fuel the passion. You will need to resolve to end the relationship and be honest with your partner about any encounters (planned or unplanned) or attempts by you or the affair partner to contact each other. Be accountable regarding your activities and be prepared to prove your trustworthiness. It may be helpful to meet together, all three of you, in order to explain to the other woman that you and your partner are back together and that you intend to make your relationship work. This is not intended to be a dramatic confrontation, but an indication to the other woman that you are committed to your partner.

Recovery from the affair depends upon several factors, such as who the other person is, how long the affair lasted, how the affair was discovered, what individual issues may exist (for example, family history of father or mother being unfaithful, history of sexual abuse, etc.), and if there is a threat that the affair is not over. Restoring trust and safety takes time. It's a gradual process usually best accomplished with the help of a trained therapist. The road to renewal may be filled with pot-holes and detours, but there's hope, especially if there's a map to follow or a guide to lead the way.

When healing from infidelity, the following strategies will be helpful:

- Together, read books about reconciliation after an affair. See the resources section for ideas.
- Write down the reasons that you still love one another. Set aside a time to share this with each other.
- Find moments to have some fun together. Make sure that, if you have children, you have some family time that reminds you of the more relaxed, trusting times from the past.
- Recall the previous times together that were positive and commit to discovering even small ways to enjoy one another again.
- Remember that verbal and nonverbal communication is vitally im-portant. Keep the lines of communication and touch open.
- Remember to show compassion. Express empathy and respect toward one another.
- When you have sex, be honest but respectful of one another's feelings and requests. The sexual relationship may be very challenging for one or both of you after the revelation of the affair. If you find that you're struggling emotionally, accept this for the present time. However, be sure to talk about the barriers to intimacy at another time.
- Don't let resentment, distrust, or anger remain so strong that you avoid a sexual relationship. Seek out someone to talk with in order to heal.
- Apologize to one another for the wounds that you've each inflicted over the course of your relationship.

Examine the following areas as they relate to you, whether you had the affair or were hurt by the affair:

- *What are our vulnerabilities?*
- *Do we have barriers between us at home?*
- *Are we opening doors to others?*
- *What are my expectations in this relationship?*
- *What are my partner's expectations?*

- *What sexual issues do we need to confront or resolve?*
- *Are we struggling with power and control issues?*
- *Do we argue endlessly about the same things?*
- *What unresolved areas of conflict are swirling around in the background of our relationship?*
- *Am I struggling with loneliness in my relationship?*

CAN'T GET ENOUGH OF THE WEB AND THE LAP DANCES!

The news is filled with examples of politicians, evangelists, and celebrities who either have been caught in a sexual scandal or have entered treatment for sexual addiction. We all probably know someone who is involved in or has been affected by his or her partner's use of Internet porn. This is a fairly recent problem in our culture. We see a greater number of couples entering therapy to deal with the issue of pornography overuse or sexual acting-out behaviors (such as frequenting strip clubs compulsively or hiring sex workers) than in the past.

It may start out innocently enough. Curiosity leads to checking out porn online that's easily accessible, inexpensive, and private. Arousal and orgasm will likely be followed by a desire to take the sexual arousal up a notch, leading some people to spend many hours and a great deal of money looking at these sites or visiting sex chatrooms. Viewing porn doesn't lead to compulsive overuse for all men and women, but Internet porn appears to have the exceptional power of false promises for gratification.

Zach and his partner came to therapy to discuss the interference of porn in their sex life. Zach explained that initially he was simply curious and searching for an avenue of excitement. He hadn't considered that he would turn to this mode of gratification, online porn sites, frequently. However, Zach found that he was repeatedly drawn to the images on the Internet because of the nature of the visual stimulation and the ease by which it could be accessed. The more time Zach spent with the computer, the less energy and sexual desire he found for his partner.

The issue of porn becomes an individual concern if it progresses to compulsive levels of use. Commonly, a person denies his or her use or dependence on the visual stimuli (or sex chatrooms, strip clubs, sex workers, etc.), but this is often short-lived and shortsighted. When a person discovers his or her partner's compulsive use of porn, it usually leads to feelings of betrayal and rejection.

Even without porn use becoming compulsive, couples rarely agree about whether chatting sexually with others online or having cybersex fit the definition of "cheating." Bader puts it well, "The issue is not that cybersex is good or bad, but that, in these cases, it has different meanings to the man engaging in it and the woman reacting to it. . . . For the man, the appeal of cybersex lies in its not being real; for women the threat lies in its reality."[2] Internet sex can be anonymous or open and interactive, but each person in the relationship needs to be able to discuss whether it crosses a line. The fantasy inherent in online sex makes this a challenging discussion. We encourage our clients to approach this subject with honesty, openness, and an empathetic ear. This can be tough. Ask each other whether the online sex enhances your own sexual relationship or detracts or greatly interferes with it.

How does someone go from simple curiosity about sex to compulsive porn use or hours spent having cybersex or setting up real-time encounters with anonymous participants? Learning to regulate and manage sexual fantasies and activities is accomplished through subtle socialization during our upbringing. We may not remember precisely how we even learned to control sexual desire and balance our innate drive with appropriate behavior. A person who has integrated sexuality into his or her emotional and intimate relationship has learned, early in life, to regulate the innate biological drive for sex. This person can have close intimate relationships and keep his or her own personal boundaries in check. His or her sex drive is accepted and integrated into the realities of the relationship.

However, the regulation of sexual desire doesn't always occur. Sometimes a person has family members who are disrespectful of others' rights or who aren't controlling their own sexual behavior. Additionally, he or she may view others as primarily sexual objects when entering puberty. Alcohol use has disinhibiting effects, which can lead to coercive and demanding sexual behavior. A person may also have experienced sexual abuse by a family member or friend that has led to a confusing array of emotions and the lowering of self-esteem. All of these influences will interfere with the integration of sexual drive into a safe and intimate relationship.

The allure of an easy, predictable, and uncomplicated "fix" is seductive to most porn users. Wendy and Larry Maltz, in their book, *The Porn Trap*, give examples of many people who have fallen into the seemingly simple trap of having their sexual needs met through porn overuse. "We may not place a personal ad that reads, 'In search of someone unreal who can meet my every sexual desire whenever and wherever without asking for anything in return,' but that's because with porn we don't have to."[3] The authors point out that most of the people they interviewed for their book had increased their porn involvement in order to deal with sexual difficulties.

SEXUAL HEALING

I've developed erectile disorder and find that I have no problem with the ED when I use porn. My partner doesn't know how much I'm looking at porn, but I don't want to give this up as it feels so good to be rid of my erectile issues when I use porn.

Dealing with sexual problems by using porn is quite common. It seems like such a simple, quick solution to the ED, but you're conditioning yourself with this behavior. It will become more and more difficult to achieve and maintain an erection with your partner as you condition your body to respond quickly, privately, and automatically to a visual image. We want to encourage you to talk with a trained therapist about this issue. Many factors need to be examined for you to gain a more intimate relationship with your partner. You'll need to explore your motivation to stop the porn. Erectile control within a real-life relationship takes self-understanding and working together with your partner on such things as types of stimulation needed and acceptance of the "ups and downs" of erections. See appendix A for more on sexual disorders for men.

Sexual acting out, such as pornography overuse or compulsive sexual behavior, is related to a "disconnect" between a person's emotional internal world and the ability to seek out appropriate sexual gratification. Sexual compulsivity is a problem of intimacy. The acting out depersonalizes sex and obscures the reality needed for a mature sexual relationship.

Lisa spoke to her therapist about her sexual compulsion. She viewed sex as a panacea for her anxieties, stress, and emotional pain. Her behavior was an expression of feelings that were usually suppressed or unacknowledged. It was very difficult for Lisa to form significant, close, and affectionate relationships because the intimacy required in a loving relationship caused her feelings of vulnerability and anxiety. Lisa's sexual acting out concealed her feelings of loneliness, sadness, anger, and fear. She found that she had developed a "relationship" with her fantasies on the Internet, sometimes spending hours looking at porn and other times losing needed sleep while chatting with strangers about sex in an adult chatroom.

There are ways to technically control Internet access so that porn sites are not available. It's important for a couple to discuss the overuse of porn, and it may help to explore the porn's emotional and sexual appeal with a trained therapist. For most people, it's intimidating to openly discuss their porn use, but it's necessary in order to seek self-understanding and to be honest about the vulnerabilities in the relationship.

 ## SEXUAL HEALING

I don't have a boyfriend so I spend a lot of time after work chatting with men online who are looking for kinky sex. I find it a real turn-on that I can entice these men and get off myself at the same time. I'm not sure I want to stop this activity. What are your thoughts about this?

You've identified very honestly that you get something from this behavior. That's an important step! We continue to do things, even destructive things, because we get something we need out of that behavior. Whether it's Internet sex or eating too much! Write down all the advantages and disadvantages of continuing your behavior. Write about how this current behavior has caused or could cause you a problem—in the past, present, and for your future. Write down your relationship goals. Do you want to eventually meet someone to live with, marry, date, or have kids with? Talk with a trusted friend or therapist about what your intimacy, sexual, or emotional fears might be. If you continue the Internet activity, you'll need to be honest with yourself that developing relationships in real time will be limited by the amount of time you spend in your virtual world.

What Porn Taught You That You Need to Re-Evaluate

Think about what you may have learned about sexuality, arousal, and gender differences from porn.

- Most porn stars have bodies that are either exceptional in appearance (penis size) or have been enhanced surgically.
- The sex in porn is usually very graphic, active, and verbal, and is all about the "come shot."
- The female genitals in porn depict the "perfect" vulva . . . symmetrical, hairless, trimmed-down labia, and juicy.
- The male in porn is usually the aggressor and has a willing partner.
- The relationship, if any is shown at all, is secondary to or absent from the sexual act.

Now think about what reality is. Your partner may not like sex with the lights on; he or she may not be comfortable with his or her appearance; the relationship is a vitally important component of sex; your partner may prefer quiet intimate sex; there may be performance issues to consider; genitals come in all sizes and shapes. Remember that porn is fantasy and not reality.

We have included some sources in the resources section of this book that explore the appeal of porn and how to heal from its impact. It's extremely important to understand this problem and not overreact to it or over-pathologize porn use. The resources we have included will help to clarify the problem, explore ways to deal with the compulsion, and build intimacy.

MOVING ACROSS THE BRIDGE

In this chapter, we've examined some tough relationship struggles, from anger and power struggles to infidelity and porn. Many times relationship challenges seem overwhelming and begin to interfere with a close and fun sexual experience. It's important to examine the difficulties, rather than tuck them away, in order to heal and learn from them. Only in this way can couples truly know one another and enjoy their sensuality.

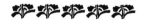

SEXERCISES

I. Consider whether you or your partner is avoiding sex. Are you avoiding each other? Do you feel like roommates? In your journal, write down some of the reasons you think you may be avoiding your partner. To help you get started, here are some possible reasons:

- I'm angry with my partner.
- I feel really bad about my body these days and don't want to be touched.
- It's been so long since we had sex that I feel awkward trying to be sexy.
- I noticed that I have developed some changes in my erections or have low desire or feel some pain with intercourse (or any other sexual difficulty).
- I don't trust my partner.
- I feel like we are just occupying space and have nothing much in common now.

If you need to talk this over with a therapist, take that step. If you can go directly to your partner, sit down together and talk about what you've discovered about yourself.

Remember to make "I feel" statements and suggest a solution, for example, "I feel scared that I'm not attractive to you. I've gotten so out of shape. I know I've been avoiding you because I don't want to be naked with you. I don't feel sexy. I can't seem to get in the mood because I feel so unattractive. Maybe we could exercise and be more health conscious together."

II. Are you and your partner arguing about who's right and who's wrong? Recall that not all problems will be resolved even with continued talking. Accepting that you are different from each other may be the wisest and most realistic path you can take.

Make a list of some of the issues that you two argue about continually, or are rehashing and getting nowhere.

Consider whether you can let some of these issues go and accept your partner with tolerance and kindness. The problems that persist may need to be taken to a trained therapist. Some issues that are commonly rehashed are discipline of the kids, in-laws, budgets, sex, time management, religion, and household chores.

III. Think about how you criticize your partner. Consider what the yearning is behind your criticism. For example, "You don't ever want to have oral sex anymore." This can be changed to express the desire, "I miss having oral sex like we used to. I really want to spice things up. Can we talk about this?" Now, try writing in your journal any criticisms that you have about your partner; write your yearning or desire, rather than a complaint.

IV. If your relationship has gone through an affair, take the time to read the material about healing from infidelity that we have recommended. Together, commit to talking about the meaning of the affair, and whether you can salvage your relationship. It's usually necessary to talk with a therapist in order to sort through the hurts and misunderstandings. Healing and rebuilding the relationship take time. If you try to rush this process, you may revisit many of the same areas later in your relationship. After there is some healing from the affair, it's helpful to write a letter to each other about the affair, whether you are the person who had the affair, or the person who was betrayed by the affair. Include your feelings and thoughts about what the affair meant to you, your own responsibility in the affair, and things you'd like to continue to work on in your relationship, etc.

V. Are you struggling with excessive use of porn? If so, take the time to understand this phenomenon. Being compulsive about porn or Internet sex chatrooms doesn't make you a "bad" or "sick" person. Make sure that you do some reading about this issue. Talk about this with someone you can trust. Seek guidance as you make the necessary repairs in your relationship. Write about how the use of porn is affecting your relationship.

VI. Let's look at obstacles to intimacy. Think about the things that you are engaged in that take you away from a fulfilling relationship. It might be avoidance of your partner, anger, endless arguing, an affair, porn overuse, constant complaining, and more. Now make a list of these obstacles in your relationship. Beside each obstacle, write down what you believe your role is in maintaining this behavior. Additionally, write down what advantage there might be in continuing the obstacle. Finally, write down what you and your partner have to gain by eliminating this obstacle. For example:

Obstacle: Constant complaining

My role: I bring up my irritation about his mother all the time. I point out her interference and want him to stop her from dominating our time.

Advantages to continuing the obstacle: I feel like things might get better if I keep telling him about it. But I also see that this keeps him on the defensive and then we argue a lot. Perhaps the arguing serves the purpose of keeping him at a distance or punishing him. Maybe I want him to feel bad and sort of suffer because he isn't solving this problem to my satisfaction.

What we have to gain by eliminating the obstacle: We would be closer and have more fun if I stopped complaining. He wouldn't be so distant and defensive with me. We might be able to problem-solve better if I wasn't always on his case. I need to stop the complaining and try to have a constructive conversation about my needs and ways that he can support me.

9

SIGHS OF PASSION

Fanning the Flame

I remember the times when we couldn't wait to see each other. I miss those days, but I'm not sure she does.

—Male, age 47

- Do you miss the more passionate moments in your relationship?
- Are you avoiding the conversations about the fading of your erotic interaction?
- Would you like to spice things up in the bedroom?
- Do you feel that you've lost your former sexual and sensual self?
- Is your partner complaining that he or she has grown tired or frustrated with the lack of sex in your relationship?

Sometimes it seems like a struggle to get to the point of having a hot, juicy sex life. But it's worth it! Sex is an integral part of life and can be pursued with a passion. Well, what's so great about sex? It improves intimacy, it relieves stress and tension, it's good for your health, it improves your quality of life, and it just plain feels great!

This chapter brings together all the aspects that have been explored in the previous chapters: the journey to understanding the sexual self. Each plank making up the bridge to sexual awareness—childhood perceptions, sexual wounds, sexual uniqueness, life-stage challenges, communication, expectations, and relationship struggles—has led to this final section of the bridge, the element of cultivating desire. Maintaining a playful and stimulating sexual relationship enhances the overall relationship. Whether the sex is hotly erotic or quietly calming, a healthy sexual relationship brings connection and warmth to a couple. But how do we keep the sexual relationship from becoming stale, obligatory, mechanical, or even nonexistent?

In therapy, Sophia spoke with a discouraged tone, explaining, "I'm afraid we've hit that point in the relationship where I just go along with sex so that Stephen won't complain or sulk. I'm so sad because I'm in my second long-term relationship and this exact thing happened in the first one!" She described feeling again the deadness of her sexual drive and a sense of obligation to have sex so that she wouldn't upset her partner. Sophia was only thirty-nine and had been with Stephen for about four years. She desperately wanted to rekindle the passion in her sexual relationship with her partner because she enjoyed the feeling of being connected emotionally. Sophia also recalled the sexual fun she and Stephen had had when first together. With the help of therapy, Sophia began to examine both her own individual triggers to desire and strategies that she and Stephen could employ to spice up the sexual relationship.

Let's look at individual triggers that can enhance sexual desire and arousal, including focusing on the senses, tuning into fantasy, choosing to be sexual, and discovering desire. As a couple, it's important to engage in strategies that invite sexual playfulness and exploration, such as making the connection, building anticipation, getting it on, and dealing with setbacks.

INDIVIDUAL TRIGGERS

Focusing on the Senses

What are the keys that unlock sexual pleasure? A great place to start is focusing on the five senses: touch, taste, hearing, sight, and smell. Life becomes so busy and packed full of things to do that many people forget about tuning into their senses and the pleasure that can be derived from them.

Certain aromas—a scent of perfume, cologne, or a candle—create a feeling of relaxation or sensuality. Perhaps the musky smell of another's

body brings up feelings and images of sexual anticipation. Hearing lyrics, rhythms, or a musical beat may quicken the pulse or just help us
unwind from a busy day. Touch of all kinds can reduce negative tension
or increase sexual tension. The stroke of another's fingers, the caressing
contact from a soft feather or warm bath—the list is endless. Tasting
deeply flavorful desserts, nibbling something decadent, or sipping a dry
buttery wine can bring the finer things of life into clearer focus after a
long day. The sight of one's partner, an erotic photograph, or one's own
aroused body may bring a feeling of pleasure.

Katie and Kyle entered therapy after Kyle discovered that Katie had begun an emotional relationship with a man at work. Kyle's responses were
all over the board—self-blame, anger at Katie, insecurity, fear, desire to
get out of the relationship before he experienced any more pain, and plans
for revenge. As the couple dealt with the fallout from Katie's emotional
entanglement, they were slowly able to examine their own emotional and
sexual relationship.

Regarding their sex life, Kyle stated that he wanted sex more often, and
Katie agreed that their sex life had become stale and routine. Katie realized that her sexual appetite seemed dulled. She explained, "I rarely feel
myself anticipating anything sexual with Kyle. I don't often think about sex
or feel internally charged up like I used to." Exploring her senses became a
key way for Katie to reawaken her sexual drive, her desire for her partner,
and her own simmering of sensual expectancy. Katie enjoyed a warm bath,
self-stimulation, the scent of candles, soft music, and having a glass of wine
before being sexual with Kyle. She also found that between their times of
sexual play, it was helpful for her to keep herself sensually charged by using
her vibrator, keeping up her exercise regimen, and reading some erotica.

Tuning into Fantasy

Fantasies are a safe and pleasurable means by which to experience
just about anything. Using fantasy is often a useful trigger for orgasm.
Stimulation starts, the tension builds, and creative personal imagery
leads the person to the intensity and pleasure of orgasm. Even without
orgasm, creating fantasies can allow a person to explore his or her sexual
energy and sensuality.

A concept that may be challenging to admit, but appears to contain a
great deal of truth, is that sexual pleasure requires a certain amount of

selfishness. Bader discusses this in his intriguing book, *Arousal: The Secret Logic of Sexual Fantasies*. "Sexual excitement also requires that we momentarily become selfish and turn away from concerns about the other's pleasure in order to surrender to our own, that we momentarily stop worrying about hurting or rejecting the other person."[1] By using masturbatory fantasy or a sexual fantasy while with a partner, people find their inhibitions easier to abandon and their arousal heightened and intensified.

If playing out a fantasy intrigues you and your partner, talk about what your roles would be and whether some things are off limits. Once you've decided who's going to be tied up and who's wearing the French maid outfit, go for it with wild abandon! Role-playing is a great way to enhance and expand your sexual repertoire without threat. Fantasy or toys . . . you decide.

So Many Toys, So Little Time   There are great websites, books, and adult-toy stores available to couples and individuals these days! We have included some in our resources section. One of our favorites is *The Many Joys of Sex Toys* by Anne Semans.[2] Here is just a sampling of some of the chapters that explain the use of the toys:

- Priming the Pump: Masturbating with a Penis Sleeve
- Missionary Zeal: Spicing Up the Missionary Position with a Cock Ring Vibrator
- Four on the Floor: Doing It Doggie-Style with a Hands-Free Vibrator
- Blow Him Away: Give a Blow Job with a Buzz
- Please Enter in the Rear: Anal Intercourse with a Dildo
- Wet and Wild: Underwater Sex Adventures

✿ SEXUAL HEALING

I'm finding my sexual desire quite deadened. As a guy, this is very disturbing to me. My physician has checked me out and everything's okay health-wise and with my testosterone. I'm in my thirties and my partner seems to be outpacing me when it comes to sexual energy. I think I'm so distracted by work stress and some family problems that I've shut down. Additionally, I'm not masturbating much because I'm so tense and distracted. Do you have any suggestions?

We would strongly encourage you to take the time to re-engage your senses and tune into your fantasies. It seems that, in an effort to survive the stress that you're under, you've turned away from pleasure, relaxation, and sensuality. Stress can kill a person's sexual energy and focus. Talk to your partner about the stress you're under, re-evaluate the wisdom of continuing to take on so much at work and with family, and take some time to be a little selfish . . . indulge your senses, get a massage, go away with your partner or alone for a weekend or an entire week, and release yourself to fantasize. Take the time to self-stimulate without the goal of orgasm, but just to feel the touch and arouse the mind with a fantasy or two.

Choosing to Be Sexual

In chapter 5, we discussed the study in which Bernie Zilbergeld asked couples over the age of forty-five to rate their sex lives.[3] He found that those who reported that their sex lives were "good" or "wonderful" were couples who made their sexual interaction a priority. These couples consisted of individuals, not surprisingly, who were dealing with a variety of aging issues. Some had physical pain, medication interference, and illness with which to contend. In spite of these challenges, the couples in this study retained their sensual interaction because they saw their sexual relationship as meaningful and worth preserving.

Individually, we can choose to treat the sexual relationship and our own individual sexuality with neglect, or we can consider that sexuality is life enhancing and relationship enriching. Consider the following questions:

- What does sex mean to me?
- What does love mean to me?
- What does not having sex (or not having much fun sex) mean to my partner?
- What does not having sex (or not having much fun sex) mean for me?
- Where will we be in five years if we don't commit to working on our sexual relationship?
- What will I/we gain by committing to exploring the sexual relationship?

So, how do we *choose* to be sexual? Pay attention to the sensual cues that trigger arousal. Indulge in some fantasies while alone. Remember hot moments of passion. Recall experiences in the past that were a turn-on and that left a feeling of warm connection or incredible sexual satisfaction. Then set aside time to be sexual or make a date for an activity that leads to erotic playfulness.

 ## SEXUAL HEALING

I'm having trouble with the notion that I need to make sex a priority in my day when I feel so fatigued and, quite frankly, angry with my partner's lack of help around the house or even much concern for my stress level! My priority right now is to stay the hell away from my partner! Okay, I got that out. . . . I do feel like we're missing out on something that used to bring us a lot of fun. Where do we start?

You can start by engaging your partner in a conversation about your needs, your stressors, and specific ways your partner can help you. Additionally, it doesn't sound like you are ready to make sex a priority right now. That's okay. Sex doesn't have to be the only way to connect with each other. Consider the many ways that the two of you have had fun together over the years. Give some thought to engaging in simple ways of bonding: dancing, going for a walk, talking over a glass of wine, hot-tubbing, sharing your day. When your relationship begins to heal and become stronger, give yourself permission to go ahead and act on any opportunity to be sexual. It might not be intercourse, but possibly mutual masturbation, oral sex, a back rub that leads to manual stimulation, or a planned make-out session. If the tension between the two of you is too negative and lasts too long, please consider therapy.

Discovering Desire

Desire is a complex concept! For males, testosterone remains consistent over time until after middle age. Therefore, for many years, desire likely continues to be steady and constant for men. However, for females, desire appears to ebb and flow, probably due to hormonal influences, and may not be something that a woman can reliably count on. However, age, conflict, illness, and stress plague both males and females, often robbing the relationship of desire.

A male with low desire will need to examine this issue with his physician. Low testosterone can be evaluated and supplemented, making a big difference in desire, energy, and mood. A physician can also determine if the lowered libido is related to medication, depression, or illness. If there's not a physical component to the loss of desire, it's important for a man to examine the other areas that may be interfering in desire. A close look at the relationship, self-esteem, trust, performance anxiety, and emotional concerns may shed light on the causes of low desire.

Females may have a tougher time teasing out the cause of low desire. The same issues that influence a male's lowered libido may also affect a woman's. Due to a woman's anatomy and cultural influences, it is often more challenging for a female to be aware of her own physiological responses to desire and arousal. Without this awareness, a female might assume that she is *not* aroused when, in fact, there may be subtle reactions to everyday experiences or specific sexual cues.

An interesting study examined female sexual arousal and genital response.[4] Women were asked to report arousal while viewing erotic material and their self-reports were correlated to the physiological measures of arousal (tested by measuring genital vasocongestion with a photoplethysmograph, a tampon-size device placed in the vagina). The women were divided into three groups: one group was instructed to attend to their genital signs of sexual arousal (vaginal lubrication, pelvic warmth, and muscular tension); a second group was instructed to attend to non-genital signs of arousal (heart rate increase, nipple erection, breast swelling, and muscular tension); and the control group was given no instructions. Both experimental groups showed high correlations between self-reports and physiological measures of arousal, while the control group showed low correlation between self-reports of arousal and the physiological measures.

The take-away message from the above study is for women to indulge their sexual awareness, be a little self-focused, and pay direct attention to their bodies. Our culture, however, does not encourage women to focus attention on their sexual self, but to focus, instead, on the partner (or even the environment and everyday stress). Pay attention to the genital and non-genital signs of arousal. Focused attention to these signals can help during everyday life and during sexual play. The more a woman feels in tune to her sexual self, the more likely she will be to awaken her erotic, playful self. When we allow ourselves to experience arousal, desire may soon follow.

COUPLES' STRATEGIES

Making the Connection

Hannah talked in therapy about her loss of libido related to pain caused by extensive endometriosis. She felt the pain had eased after surgery to remove the endometriosis, her uterus, and her ovaries. However, she didn't feel much of a connection to her former sexual drive or to her partner, Hank. Hank, usually very passive, was beginning to become unhappy with the lack of sex in their relationship. He was careful not to blame Hannah, but wanted to do something to feel close and sexual again. Hannah was on a low dose of hormone replacement following the hysterectomy, and this was helping her regain her libido. However, she talked about being afraid of intercourse, as she'd experienced a great deal of pain with the endometriosis. Fortunately, Hannah felt motivated to work at regaining their sexual relationship.

The therapist talked to them about their individual triggers and encouraged them to focus on their senses and their fantasies. Hannah liked the idea of paying more attention to her own sexual awareness through focusing on her genital and non-genital sensations related to fantasies. After discussing their daily and weekly routine, Hank and Hannah determined that they had little time for connection. Between work, the household chores, two kids, Hannah's nursing program, and Hank's love of hunting, they seemed to be going in opposite directions most of the times. Once they explored their schedules, Hank determined that he could make some changes to his daily routines and hunting trips to spend more time with Hannah and the kids. Hannah also decided to slow things down a bit with her nursing program so that she had more time for herself, their relationship, and the kids.

Physical and emotional connection is vital in order to fan the flames. In therapy, we often hear clients talk about feeling too tired or too distant to engage sexually with their partners. It's understandable that someone might feel that there is a huge chasm to leap from being "mom and dad" or "the Smiths" or "the dentist and the teacher" to a hot, turned-on couple!

What can we do to make the connection? Like Hannah and Hank, spending time exploring the routines or schedules of everyday life can reveal possible barriers to connecting. We need to be honest about whether there are things on our to-do lists that create a gulf between our partner and us. Are those things there to help us avoid intimacy? Is there underlying conflict or resentment that needs to be voiced and discussed, perhaps with a therapist? Are there fears about becoming more sexual? A sexual connection brings with it a great deal of fun and playfulness; however, we may not always feel deserving of pleasure. If there is resistance or hesitancy due to emotional barriers, it's vital to openly discuss this as a couple.

Make touching a priority in the relationship. All kinds of touch: comforting, companionate, playful, affectionate, and erotic. Without frequent touch, sensual and sexual encounters can become awkward. Couples who continue to touch each other often find they are able to problem-solve more easily in everyday situations because they feel connected and safe.

Building Anticipation

In therapy, we hear about the struggle to find sexuality in long-term relationships. Sometimes couples can recall a time when the intensity of desire was palpable, but later lament that they can no longer effortlessly move to a sexual relationship. Too many chores, children, and challenges have crept into bed with them. We need to allow some simmering of sexual anticipation before moving to the erotic. Building this anticipation is a lot like visualizing a repeat trip to a favorite restaurant. Just remembering the familiar and tantalizing sights, aromas, and tastes creates expectation and hope for satisfaction. Just as one dreams of this tempting culinary experience, visualization of a favorite sexual encounter can create an eagerness for more.

 SEXUAL HEALING

I'm really trying to give myself some time to think about my sexual turn-ons, but I find that I have no idea how to do this. I think my life is so busy that I just go through the motions of each day and suddenly I'm home with my partner and not really ready to be sexual. I know I need to spice things up! Help!

Allow yourself to think of ways that you might turn up the heat through-
out your day. Notice the feel of your sweater against your skin. Think
about a time that was especially exciting sexually, and just daydream
about that during your lunch hour. Perhaps pay attention to signs of
arousal—genital and muscular tension, heavier breathing, lubrication,
and other physical sensations—as you remember a sexy interaction.
Then call and leave a message for your partner including your current
fantasy, or a remembered sexual encounter, or what you'd like to try
tonight when you get home from work. Text message a tantalizing line
or two to your partner and give some hints about what he or she can
anticipate for the evening or the "coming" weekend.

Once you and your partner are together, take any opportunity that seems
welcome to make that sexy connection: enjoy a sensual kiss, give a back
rub, offer a massage, or caress your partner's inner thigh or lower back.
Go dancing together and immerse yourselves in the musical beat. Perhaps
leave some clothes behind in the car to surprise your partner as you sway
closely on the dance floor. Explore an adult-toy store together, whispering
about the exciting things that the two of you might do with some of the toys.
Try something new: a sensual new lubricant, a fun vibrator, some light re-
straints, a blindfold, whatever looks like fun and that you both agree on.

❀❀❀

The saying "use it or lose it" is an encouragement to play sexually as
often as possible. The purpose of this is to keep the body, genital tissues,
hormones, and the mind juicy and charged as long as possible. It's a really
great idea to take some time out of the day, perhaps on a weekend afternoon alone, to do a little self-pleasuring. One of the most helpful ways that
a person can learn about their desire, arousal, and orgasm triggers is to
self-stimulate without any inhibitions or time restrictions. This takes some
planning, so make sure important things are in place: privacy, toys, candles,
music, some erotic reading. Later you can share the afternoon delight with
your partner by recounting the buildup, the fantasy, and the incredible finish! Or promise your partner a repeat performance for the next time!

Read or watch something a little (or a lot!) racy to build anticipation
for a hot sexual encounter. We have listed some reading material in the
resources section of this book. Together, read an erotic book, enjoying the narrative and dialogue, but also enjoying one another's sexual

response to the fantasy. Take turns writing your own erotica. Write a line or two and then hand it off to your partner to write more. As you send it back and forth, the excitement can build to an intense climax, or just toss the writing aside and act it out! Read a sex-advice book or article aloud that gives hints to overcome inhibitions or suggestions for new techniques. Some couples enjoy watching an erotic film together because it can be stimulating physically and to the imagination.

 ## SEXUAL HEALING

My partner wants to try some new things in the bedroom, and I'm really feeling shy about it. We've talked about going to an adult-toy store or reading erotica. I think I'm way too inhibited to try this stuff! But my partner isn't! I feel kind of pushed to go along with his fantasy. I think he thinks that I'll just come alive with desire and be a hot babe if I try new things. What do I do?

First, it would be helpful to talk openly with your partner about your fears and your shyness. He needs to be given the opportunity to hear your fears. Don't feel that you have to go along with his fantasies and ignore your own feelings. Second, you can look online at adult toys and erotic films to see if anything there looks interesting and not too intimidating. You might do this alone so that you don't feel the pressure from your partner to try something that looks out of your comfort zone. Third, look back at the questions under the heading, "Choosing to Be Sexual." You and your partner can talk about these issues from the standpoint of exploring what sexual experimentation means to both of you. It may be that you're shy due to a family background of shame or inhibition. Or it may be that your idea of sex, love, and sexual experimentation are just different from your partner's ideas. You don't have to agree with each other on this. However, you might consider one of the toys featured in an online store, a new sexual position, or reading a sex-advice article in a magazine together. If you try something new and don't really like it, just tell your partner that it's not for you. Keep yourself open to new ideas and experiences, but don't make yourself over just to please someone else.

Getting It On!

It *does* look great in the movies, doesn't it? The thrusting, throbbing, breathless entanglements depicted in fiction are certainly more erotic than most average couples' experiences. But sexual encounters in long-term relationships don't have to consist of the same old technique, position, and lukewarm finish.

Good sex needs to be worth having. What does it take to make getting it on worthwhile? One way to examine sexual needs is to look at fantasies, exploring what the fantasies may say about erotic desires. What is evocative in your fantasy and how can that translate to actual sex: more moaning, more dirty talking, less verbalizing, different types of stimulation, changing positions, mutual masturbation, longer-lasting encounters, more foreplay, more oral stimulation, less rubbing? It's helpful to think this through and then talk to your partner about it.

Kiss Me Quick! Remember when you and your partner were dating? You were kissing all the time . . . kissing goodnight, kissing hello, kissing in the front seat, kissing in the backseat! Think not only about how much time you spent kissing, but the reaction of your body when you experienced those long, passionate kisses. More than likely your breath and heart rate quickened. If you're male, you possibly became erect, and if you're female, your genitals probably became engorged and lubricated. There was definitely a reaction in your body that began with a kiss.

Is kissing a long-lost memory in your relationship? When was the last time you kissed your partner with passion? How much of your lovemaking sessions are devoted to "making out"? It seems that kissing is usually a primary part of foreplay and lovemaking at the beginning of the relationship, but then it tends to disappear as the relationship ages. Try adding more kissing to your sexual encounters. Kiss your partner longingly in the kitchen when you want to say, "Come hither . . ." or try more kissing with foreplay. It could be exciting to kiss with your eyes open, or right at the moment of orgasm.

Do Me Quick! Does sex always have to be a well-orchestrated dance? Absolutely not. Sex can be a quickie in the backseat of a car, a hot entanglement in the walk-in closet, or a rendezvous in the hotel shower; these encounters can be a wonderful release.

Hot August Night What do we need in order to turn up the heat? How can we make our encounters sizzle? Most females need clitoral stimulation in order to feel adequate arousal to achieve orgasm. Clitoral massage can be done orally, manually, with a penis (erect or non-erect), or with a vibrator or other toys. Some women enjoy rubbing against their partner's body, clothed or unclothed. Remember, if you don't have orgasms with intercourse alone, that's pretty normal! Some sexual positions are more conducive to clitoral contact than others and we've explained a few of those in the section below, "Night Moves . . . or Any Time of Day."

Sometimes anxiety or fears get in the way of allowing the body to build to sufficient levels of arousal. This may lead to delayed ejaculation or erectile failure in males or anorgasmia (absent orgasm) or even physical discomfort in females. It can be helpful to think of arousal as ascending intensity with a "10" being the highest point, or orgasm. Paying attention to the body's responses, both in self-stimulation and partner-stimulation, can provide much-needed information regarding the increasing stages of arousal. For many males, it's important not to transition to intercourse until reaching an "8" or "9" on the ascending scale. If a man moves to intercourse too soon, he may not have received the type or amount of stimulation that he needs for orgasm.

Some females can move too quickly to intercourse when they are trying to please a partner or feeling anxiety about the time it takes to experience full arousal. It's important to request what is needed: the type or duration of stimulation, the right positions, or perhaps more pillows for added comfort or angling.

Night Moves . . . or Any Time of Day Some heterosexual intercourse positions may make orgasm more attainable for women, as advised in the Berman and Berman book, *For Women Only*.[5] These include:

- Missionary position with the woman's pelvis tilted up, perhaps with a pillow. This angles the woman for G-spot stimulation. It also helps the woman angle herself so that the clitoris and labia will receive more friction.
- The woman can have her partner lie across her body, shifting his pelvis forward, so that the base of his penis makes contact with the clitoris. The motion is then a rocking, back and forth movement. The female leads the upward motion, while the male leads the downward motion.
- The woman-on-top position allows the female to adjust her pelvis and control the friction of the base of the penis as it rubs against the labia

and clitoris. This position can also allow for deep thrusting, which can lead to stimulation of the cervix and a pelvic floor orgasm.

- Using Kegel exercises, or pelvic muscle flexing, during intercourse can give a woman greater friction against the partner's penis and lead to stimulation of the part of the clitoris that lies against the vaginal wall.

Other night moves include (these don't necessarily aid in clitoral stimulation):

- Rear-entry position is when the man faces the woman's back. The woman might be kneeling or lying on her stomach, hips raised slightly.
- The side-to-side position includes the man and woman lying beside each other, either face to face or in the rear-entry position. This position can be helpful for prolonged sex and hands are usually free for clitoral stimulation.
- A variation on the man-on-top position is when the woman lies on the edge of the bed, feet on the floor, while the man is standing. The woman can also lie on the edge of a table or the office desk.
- The woman-on-top position can also include the man sitting on a chair with the woman on his lap, face-to-face.

There are many variations and great DVDs to illustrate these positions. We've listed some of these in our resources section. Of course, you can add toys or creative moves to any of the above techniques, as well as variations for same-sex couples.

✿ SEXUAL HEALING

My partner has occasional erectile failure and I'm not sure how I can help him. I know he's embarrassed and self-conscious about it. He used to just get discouraged and turn away from me when he couldn't keep his erection. Now we're trying to talk more about what he needs, but it's so difficult for us!

It's great that you two are trying to talk about this issue. It isn't easy to discuss; that's true for most people with any sexual disorder. Remember

*to keep in mind the good-enough sex model—that ALL sexual encoun-
ters won't be 100 percent satisfactory.[6] So be patient as your partner is
figuring out what he needs in order to keep his erection. Try all kinds
of experimentation with sexual play and don't worry about the "ups
and downs" of his erections. This is normal. Talk to your partner about
what sorts of touch—rubbing, manual, oral—he might want to try. Take
an evening or afternoon just to explore different modes of touch and
arousal. Look at this time as an experiment and enjoy learning about
your partner's body. If it doesn't lead to intercourse that is satisfying for
you, just take an alternative route, such as using a vibrator or receiving
oral stimulation. Remember to talk to your partner about what you'd
both like for "afterplay," regardless of whether the erection lasts.*

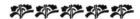

Dealing with Setbacks

In long-term relationships, partners recall the times when both made
every effort to emotionally connect and set aside time for sensual dates.
All too often, these close times get pushed aside for the mundane things
of life.

Wendy and William began to look at their emotional and sexual distance
when their children were both away at college. They remembered a time
that they'd been very sexually involved with each other and devoted to
spending time together. Wendy explained, "I had lost a lot of weight after
starting an exercise program and felt really good about my body. William
had been diagnosed with hypertension, and he made changes to his diet
and work schedule so that he could relax more, exercise, and slow down.
Now we've both fallen back into those poor habits of being too busy for
each other, being too tired to exercise, and eating out a lot. But in the
past three years, with the kids away at college, it seems like we need to be
enjoying this time more!" William agreed with Wendy.

Together they made a list of things they could do to ensure more emotional closeness: spend time in the hot tub talking at the end of the day,
begin to exercise to bolster energy, schedule date night at least every
other week, and arrange a getaway twice a year to a romantic spot. However, when it came to their sex life, they seemed unsure about how to
rekindle the passion and desire.

It's important to work simultaneously on both the emotional and sexual relationship. As we've pointed out, becoming a caring and compassionate couple will not necessarily generate erotic desire. Take time out every week or two to enjoy giving and receiving sensual massage or a sensate focus session with intercourse off limits. Explore new positions, read erotic literature, or try something that's a little edgy and different. If too much time elapses and neither partner is moving toward the other, it may be time to visit with a sexuality or relationship therapist in order to explore the resistance.

✷ SEXUAL HEALING

I read recently that it's a good idea to take a break from sex sometimes and just enjoy the sensuality of touch. My partner and I are in a bit of a disagreement about how to carry this out. She's interested in trying this to see what she feels like without the pressure to have intercourse. But I have to admit, as a guy, I'm pretty sure that if we get started with a lot of touching and massaging, I'm going to be frustrated if we don't have sex!

We've heard this more than once from males! It's normal and healthy to have a sexual appetite and to desire intercourse. The idea of having sessions without intercourse as the end goal is what sensate focus was based on. This can alleviate performance anxiety, help an individual learn all sorts of important things about his or her body and its responses, and allow for new paths of pleasure to be created. So how about sex taking a holiday? Perhaps that can be an encouragement—just to take a little holiday from the usual. If there's a disagreement about this exercise, allow the partner who wants to take the holiday to enjoy the sensuality of caresses and massage. And remember, there are always the other forms of stimulation to orgasm—oral, manual, rubbing, etc. Be sure to talk to each other about what your goals are with this exercise.

MOVING ACROSS THE BRIDGE

The bridge to sexual awareness and enriching sensual interaction is an important structure to explore and to strengthen. We've crossed the bridge to sexual awareness. By using the techniques of individual triggers and couples' strategies, along with lots of communication, you will be on your way to hotter, sexier hookups. The next two chapters can assist you in investigating your sexual self as you have conversations with your physical and mental health-care providers.

🕏🕏🕏🕏🕏

SEXERCISES

I. Take some time to fantasize. Put in a DVD that turns you on or read some sizzling erotica. Simmer your sexual imaginings and physical sensations. Become aware of your genital and non-genital arousal—heavier breathing, quickening heart rate, erection or lubrication, muscular tension, etc. Pay special attention to what forms of stimulation are arousing. Do you enjoy single stimulation or multiple stimulation (nipple *and* clitoris, penis *and* perineum)? Would you like to have your partner talking dirty or moaning? Do you think you would be aroused by seeing your partner masturbate? Does pacing make a difference to you in your sexual response? What are some of the triggers for your particular orgasm pattern? Think about what turns you on and gets you to that "point of no return" in your fantasies. Share this information with your partner. Explore whether these avenues to pleasure are as effective in reality or are best left to fantasy.

II. Pelvic floor exercises, sometimes called Kegel exercises, are used to strengthen the pelvic floor muscles and connective tissue. These muscles act to support internal organs, enhance sexual function, and provide closure of the anal and urethral sphincters.

In an article on her website, Talli Rosenbaum, a urogynecological physiotherapist and certified sex counselor, points out that strengthening the pelvic floor muscles can improve blood flow to the genitals, which can enhance sexual response.[7] Rosenbaum discusses the many other reasons to strengthen these muscles (preventing and treating urinary incontinence, prolapse of the bladder, uterus, or rectum, and back pain, etc.). Rosenbaum's article explains how to identify if you are doing the Kegel exercise correctly. Her advice is to insert a finger into the vagina, tighten the muscles around the finger, take a deep breath, and when exhaling, use your vaginal muscle to squeeze your finger. Simultaneously, pull the navel in toward the spine.

We have included a website in the resources guide that provides a "pelvic floor educator" that may help you teach yourself the correct Kegel exercise. This device includes an indicator wand that will move down, away from the body, when the exercise is done correctly. We are not endorsing this product, but are suggesting you take a look at it and talk with your physician about its usefulness.

Rosenbaum also indicates in the above article that men may find that building the pelvic floor will improve erection and help in controlling the timing of ejaculation. Rosenbaum suggests that males place a finger on the perineum (the area of skin between the scrotum and anus). At this point, the man will tighten the anal muscles as though trying to prevent gas from escaping. The man will then inhale and exhale while squeezing. Again, he is to pull the navel in toward the spine, thus lifting the perineum.

When these muscles have been identified, it's a good idea to contract them during regular activities, such as coughing or sneezing, or when lifting or pulling heavy objects. During sexual activity, consciously contracting and relaxing these muscles can help with blood flow to the genital area, thus stimulating and enhancing sexual response.

III. You've probably heard of Tantra. It's a very old spiritual practice, similar to yoga, that originated in ancient India. Tantra takes many years of commitment and study; however, we can use some of the tenets of Tantra to enrich our sex lives and get a taste of enlightenment with some of the techniques. Dr. Judy Kuriansky states the word Tantra comes from an ancient language meaning "expansion through awareness."[8] The purpose of Tantra is to help us experience the intensity of our feelings and allow more potential for pleasure. The technique of Tantric sex allows us to feel sensually, with a greater passion.

Tantric sex is a spiritual experience that lets us be present not only with our partner, but with ourselves. Tantra makes use of the yin/yang qualities in all of us. Every individual has a unique mix of both masculine and feminine qualities. Tantric philosophy requires that we seek to become balanced in both the male and the female, allowing ourselves to become integrated or unified.

As another option for experiencing sexual pleasure, Tantra has been an alternative for those who are disabled and challenged in the area of sex. In general, we see sex as beginning with excitement and culminating with orgasm. Tantric sex tells us to slow the process down in order to remain in the moment, allowing us to hold on to the sexual energy instead of the energy being "spent" with the climax, or orgasm. As we've pointed out, Western sex tends to be goal-oriented and failure to orgasm is often seen as an embarrassment or disappointment. Tantric sex, on the other hand, takes the pressure off the goal of orgasm, offering us an opportunity to connect with our partner or ourselves on a much deeper level.

What are some of the techniques we can use to get a feel for Tantric sex? Here are some ideas, but be sure to check out the resources in the back of the book to get more information and in-depth explanations of Tantric sex.

- Control your breath. When you exhale for a longer period than you inhale, it tends to relax you.
- Breathing with your partner helps you to connect. Sit cross-legged, facing your partner and looking into each other's eyes. Try to breathe with each other, getting into the same breathing rhythm. Try to sit with this connection for a period of time.
- Switch so that you are breathing opposite each other. Exhale while your partner inhales, and inhale while your partner exhales.
- Incorporate your senses . . . candlelight, appropriate music, soft pillows, or whatever it is that you find sensual.
- Resist the urge to breathe quickly when stimulating each other. Heavy breathing invites arousal, moving you toward orgasm. Take long, deep breaths from your belly, exhaling slowly. During foreplay, try using the above techniques of matching your breath to your partner's, or breathing alternately—as you inhale, your partner exhales. This moves the sexual energy back and forth and connects you to your partner.

IV. Talk to your partner about trying new positions, if this interests you. In the resources section, we have listed some great websites with DVDs that will explicitly show new and exciting sexual positions and techniques. Together, watch or read the instructions and enjoy experimenting with the new pathways to pleasure.

V. Be sure to read "Pillow Talk" in chapter 6. That section gives some fun verbal and nonverbal ways to stay connected and sensual in your relationship. Here are a few more:

- Go ahead and get a little something sexy to surprise your partner, either wearing it under your clothes and out in public, or slipping into it at bedtime.
- Using something light and sexy, loosely tie your partner to the bedposts. Then kiss and caress every inch of his or her body, except the genitals.
- Make up a basket of your partner's favorite wine, appetizers, and chocolates, and add a new toy or lubricant as a surprise.
- Building to orgasm can be enjoyed very slowly if you back away from the intensity of arousal. You can do this by starting and stopping the stimulation just before orgasm, over and over again.
- Mutual masturbation incorporates the visual sight of your partner's arousal and also the intensity that comes from your own self-knowledge about your body.
- Keep your clothes on for a make-out session and then undress each other.
- Give your partner a lap dance. If you feel intimidated about this, take a belly dancing class or pole dancing class.
- Get it on in an unusual place for the two of you . . . the bathtub, the car, the deck, the garage, the kitchen floor, the shower.

III

IS ANYONE LISTENING?

When we went through my cancer treatment, I felt that any questions we asked the professionals about sex were met with a bit of embarrassment or that we were cut off and ignored.

—Female, age 58

10

TALKING WITH YOUR THERAPIST

- Do you feel comfortable bringing up the topic of sex in therapy?
- Does your therapist bring up the subject of sex?
- Do you feel like you or your therapist is avoiding the topic of sex?
- Do you have trouble broaching the subject of sex in couples therapy?
- Are you a therapist who is having trouble discussing sexual issues in therapy?

This book is considered a self-help book, but it's not intended to take the place of good ol' face-to-face therapy. If the need is to find a therapist who can help make sense out of life and guide a person through difficult situations, we want to help with that pursuit. This chapter will cover several aspects of the therapeutic relationship, including how to find a therapist who can help, what to expect in therapy, and how to bring up those hard-to-discuss topics.

SEXUAL HEALING

Help! I went to see a therapist, and every time I brought up my sex life, he changed the subject! This is a huge issue for me and my partner and

I really need to talk about it. I stopped seeing the therapist and still have no one to talk to about my feelings. I don't know what to do. I feel too ashamed to bring it up again to a therapist. Obviously, I should never have brought it up.

This must have been so frustrating for you! There are therapists out there who can help you get some resolution to your problem; it just takes some footwork to find the right one. Be sure you tell the therapist as early as the initial phone call that your problem is of a sexual nature, so she can refer you to someone else if she doesn't feel competent in that area. If the therapist says she doesn't feel able to treat sexual issues, ask if she knows anyone in the area who might specialize in sex therapy. Another option is to check with your physician, nurse practitioner, gynecologist, or urologist for referrals. You can also go online to www.aasect.org to find a certified sex therapist in your area. Don't give up! Your issue is a legitimate issue for therapy and you deserve help with your problem.

In chapter 1, we gave an example of a couple who came to therapy and told the therapist that they hadn't been asked about sex by their past therapist. The couple had also not brought up the topic of sex in their current therapy sessions. This has been a common complaint in our private practice. If sex is an issue that is affecting a person's life, not only should it be brought up in therapy, it should be dealt with in a sensitive, understanding manner.

FINDING THE RIGHT THERAPIST

An acquaintance called the office of our private practice one day and asked for advice about finding a therapist. She was frantic, saying, "I'm trying to find a good therapist and I have no idea what I'm looking for! How can I find the right therapist who can deal with my particular problem? What do all those initials mean after their names? I'm overwhelmed just by looking up "therapist" and "counselor" in the phone book!" Let's look at the differences in a therapist's therapeutic orientation, type of degree, and specialties.

Therapeutic Orientation

Therapists have different theoretical orientations, or ways of conceptualizing their client's problems. There is no incorrect orientation; however, it's important to choose a therapist who has an orientation that's in line with the client's way of thinking. It's helpful if a client and therapist discuss initially, even in a phone call, what orientation the therapist uses. Here is a description of the orientations used by most therapists.

Note: *It's important to keep in mind that none of these styles of therapy are right or wrong. Therapists see problems and their solutions in different ways. It's only wrong when a therapist and client aren't seeing eye-to-eye regarding the approach.*

Cognitive/Behavioral Therapy Cognitive/behavioral therapy deals with a client's thinking patterns, with the goal of changing negative thought patterns and behaviors in order to manage symptoms and improve the quality of life. Homework and assignments outside of the therapy room are usually involved.

Interpersonal Therapy Interpersonal therapy focuses on current life and relationships. Current problems are rooted in previous relationships. The goal is to use insight to identify and resolve life problems and build on the person's strengths.

Psychoanalysis Psychoanalysis sees past conflicts as the key to current problems. The client explores unconscious motivations and earlier patterns of resolving issues. Psychoanalysis involves frequent sessions and is long-term.

Couples Therapy Couples go to therapy together to try to work through specific problems, learn better ways to communicate, and problem-solve some of the issues in their relationship.

Family Therapy Family therapy treats more than one member of a family at the same time. The therapist sees the problems as belonging to a *system*, and if one member changes, the system will be affected and change will occur for the family.

Psychodynamic Psychotherapy This orientation is based on the idea that our behavior is determined by our past experiences, genetic makeup, and current issues. Emotions and unconscious motivation have a significant impact on behavior.

Kevin came to therapy to learn to manage rapid ejaculation at the advice of his physician. Kevin did all the footwork and found a therapist he felt he could work well with, although he really never knew about the differences in a therapist's theoretical orientation. Kevin was the kind of person who focused on solutions, so the background of the problem didn't really matter to him. The therapist he found was a female, because he said he felt more comfortable talking to females, and she had a counseling degree, which he felt was perfect for his problem. He didn't know that she tended to be more psychodynamic in orientation. Several weeks into the therapy, Kevin told his physician that therapy wasn't working for him because all the therapist wanted to talk about was his past. The physician advised him to talk to his therapist about the orientation problem, and together Kevin and his therapist were able to find another therapist in the same office who worked in the way Kevin was comfortable. Kevin was able to learn new sexual techniques from a certified sex therapist, who tended to be more cognitive/behavioral in orientation.

Types of Degree

When looking for a therapist, there are all kinds of letters behind the names of the different providers. What do all these letters stand for? Most importantly, a competent therapist will have a master's or doctorate degree in the field of mental health, and be licensed or certified by the authorities in that field. A therapist should have a current license and be in good standing with the licensing board. Depending on the state the client resides in, the initials behind the therapist's name might be slightly different.

Licensed Professional Counselor   This mental health provider has at least a master's degree in the field of psychology or counseling. Check to be sure the counselor has had supervised clinical experience as part of his or her training, as books and classwork cannot substitute for clinical practice in psychotherapy. Some initials you might see are LPC, MFCC, AAPC, or NCC.

Clinical Psychologist   A psychologist in most states has a doctorate in the field of psychology or counseling. Again, be sure the psychologist has had supervised clinical experience. Psychologists are licensed in clinical psychology. Initials you might see are PhD, PsyD, or EdD.

Clinical Social Worker   Clinical social workers often have at least a master's degree in the field of social work. They have specialized clinical training; initials you might see are LCSW.

Marriage and Family Therapists   Marriage and family therapists have at least a master's degree and have clinical experience with marriage and family therapy. MFT is an initial found by their names.

Specialties

A therapist should have an understanding of the issue that brought the person into therapy. Therapists may have areas of specialization or certification, such as couples, depression, eating disorders, sex, or anxiety. Some therapists are more general in focus, so they may deal with many kinds of issues. Usually asking is the only way to know what a therapist's specialties are, and the sooner the better. The best time to ask this question is when the client makes the initial phone call to set up an appointment. As a therapist, there is nothing more disappointing than to find out that you can't help after a person pours his or her heart out to you. A client should always ask what kind of experience a therapist has had with the problem the client is trying to resolve.

A certified sex therapist is one type of specialist; individuals with this certification are trained in treating the psychological and behavioral aspects of sexual concerns and disorders. Their background and licensure will be in mental health, medicine, or social work.

Whether considering orientation, degree, or specialty, the most important aspect of therapy is the relationship the client has with the therapist. Therapy is a much richer experience than just learning to change behavior or problem-solve situations. A client should pay attention to his or her gut feeling when seeking a therapist. If it doesn't feel right, it probably isn't the right therapist. A therapist should appreciate that he or she isn't the right provider for every person, and be understanding and respectful if the client doesn't feel a connection. There are factors to consider in a therapist-client relationship, such as the way each interacts with the other and the personalities of both parties involved. A therapist should never make you feel guilty for not feeling a therapeutic connection and seeking that connection elsewhere.

 SEXUAL HEALING

Help! I've been to several sessions with a new therapist and just didn't feel a connection! Her style was direct and confrontational, which might be all right for some people, but not for me! What do I do? How will I know it's a good match?

When you go to therapy, it's important that you feel comfortable. Not every therapist and client pairing is a good fit. Do talk to the therapist

you are seeing, as it may be a therapeutic issue that you need to process.
A therapist shouldn't try to convince you to stay, but help you figure out
what you need to do and how to find the right solution.

✿ ✿ ✿

Therapy should feel comfortable and safe. Ask yourself the following
in the first session:

- Am I feeling listened to?
- Am I feeling like the therapist is paying attention?
- Am I okay with the therapist's reaction to my information?
- Am I feeling safe?

A therapist should readily discuss such factors as fees, missed sessions, length of the session, treatment, and what goals the client wants to
work on in therapy. These matters need to be discussed early in therapy,
as early as the first session. The client should feel comfortable bringing
up and discussing any relevant issue.

Websites for Finding a Therapist

- www.aasect.org (to find a certified sex therapist, counselor, or
  educator)
- www.apahelpcenter.org/articles/article.php?id=51
- www.helpguide.org/mental/psychotherapy_therapist_counseling.htm
- www.mayoclinic.com/health/mental-health/MH00008
- www.nami.org

WHAT TO EXPECT IN THERAPY

Talk therapy generally consists of a client sharing his or her life with the
therapist, using communication to help the therapist understand what
problems the client would like to work on in the therapeutic setting. In
addition to sharing day-to-day life, the therapist will want to know feelings,
behaviors, dreams, fantasies, and wishes, both positive and negative.

There are a few important points that are crucial to keep in mind
about expectations for therapy. First, therapy is not always a pleasant experience. When a client gets into the process of therapy, he or she may

be discussing bad memories, faulty patterns and behaviors, and difficult feelings. This is "grist for the therapy mill." In other words, if going to therapy makes the client feel miserable, it's important that the therapist is made aware so that adjustments to therapy can be made, if needed. Sometimes pain and hurt simply need to be felt and "sat with" for a time. A good therapist can monitor this and know what is helpful and what is not productive. Secondly, change is slow and difficult. The client can mark his or her progress in therapy by looking at improvements such as mood changes, feeling more connected with others, or handling situations in a better manner. When it comes to entrenched problems, it's important to take into consideration that it took many years to learn these maladaptive ways of thinking and behaving. As a result, it will take more than a couple of weeks to unlearn them.

A therapist can't, and shouldn't, tell a client what to do. Therapists act as guides, helping their clients discover many different aspects of themselves. This self-discovery helps a client understand what facets need to be different and how to go about changing them. Only the client can make the changes necessary to live a happy and productive life.

HOW ABOUT WHEN SEX IS THE ISSUE?

When a client sees a therapist about a particular problem, it's important to share what that problem is early in the treatment. The reason is to be sure that the therapist is competent in treating that specific issue. Even if the therapist has expertise in couples therapy or marriage and family therapy, his or her training may not be adequate in the area of sex. If the therapist does not feel competent addressing the client's sexual concerns, it becomes necessary for the therapist and client to consider a referral to a therapist who can treat the client's issue. Therapists come across issues that they have no expertise in from time to time, and are generally happy to refer. Remember—for the most part, therapists want to help and will do what is necessary to be sure clients receive the help they need.

If sex is the issue, it's essential to find a therapist who is willing to broach the subject. Due to a therapist's own set of characteristics, there may be reasons the therapist has difficulty discussing sex. If your therapist can't have a conversation about sexual matters, that generally doesn't have anything to do with the client. Therapists are human, and as a result have their own issues. The only way to know if they are on board with the whole sex conversation is to ask! The client has a right to get his or her psychological needs met in therapy, and the right to talk about sex with someone who understands the topic.

Should I Go to Couples or Individual Therapy?

When sexual or relationship concerns are a problem, it's hard not to see the issue as a "couple" issue. The best-case scenario is that the couple be seen in therapy together. In our practice, it's common that one of the members of the couple doesn't want to go to therapy for various reasons. How does that work for the couple? When the couple is working on sexual matters we encourage both partners to attend, but we can work with the individual if that's the best we can do. Sometimes, the other member of the couple realizes that his or her partner is changing and decides to get in on the action—joining the partner in therapy. Don't stay away from healing just because your partner is uncomfortable! Sexual health is a good thing in so many ways; it's worth the work and effort.

Okay, I Found a Therapist, Now What?!

As we mentioned above, the therapist should have discussed "housekeeping" issues such as fees, missed appointments, and frequency early in the therapy. Now it's time to get down to business because there is a therapeutic relationship to establish. Most people don't walk into a therapist's office with feelings of trust for the therapist right off the bat.

There may be positive feelings about the therapist, and that's a good thing. But therapy goes to some pretty scary, vulnerable places at times, so good feelings really aren't enough. Building trust becomes an important part of therapy. As with other relationships, it's okay to throw an issue out there, get a feel for how the therapist handles the issue, then go a little deeper into the matter when the therapist treats it with care and empathy.

Opening up can be frightening, especially when there are secrets that have been kept for a period of time or there are shameful feelings involved. When we feel like there is something we're hesitant to talk about in therapy, we have to remember that the things we *don't* address in the therapy room are often the ones that *need* to be addressed.

Note: *If you have the feeling that you can't discuss an issue, talk to your therapist about feeling that there is something you can't bring up in therapy. Let your therapist help you process this feeling so it doesn't continue to stand in the way of getting all you can from the therapeutic process.*

IF YOU ARE A THERAPIST

Most people who become therapists already have an empathic, warm way of interacting with other people, as well as an understanding of various personalities and their characteristics. Sex is as much a part of people as are their personality characteristics, family origins, or current situations. Graduate school programs might not have addressed human sexuality in the curriculum or clinical training, let alone provided instruction regarding how to talk to someone with erectile dysfunction or shame about masturbation.

If sex was not a part of our therapist training, we must consider seeking out continuing education on this subject. Every single person is a sexual being, and if we address only part of the person, and leave this important piece out, we are ignoring a vital aspect of that person as a whole. We have to consider our own biases and issues, and think about dealing with them in our own personal therapy. It's important to keep in mind that as therapists we are human and will have weaknesses; however, it's imperative to know what they are and deal with them accordingly. Oftentimes, we forget or feel too busy to seek supervision or consult with a colleague. These are viable options and, as therapists, we should be utilizing them more frequently than we do.

Keep in mind that our clients bring up the tougher issues when we have already established a solid, trusting relationship, so we have to be very sensitive and considerate of this trust when the tougher issue is one we struggle with ourselves. When confronted with something we struggle with as individuals, supervision or consultation is a must, in order to act in the client's best interest. It's important to remember that not every client is heterosexual. Try not to assume, as clients may have difficulty bringing up the topic of orientation or transgendered issues.

The goal is to be helpful to our clients. We have the education, empathy, and desire to help others, so why not be sure we can address every aspect of the person, and not just bits and pieces? To take this even further, this means that when it comes to sex, we should be part of an interdisciplinary team, as there are aspects of sexuality that should be considered besides the psychological component. Working with physicians, gynecologists, urologists, oncologists, urogynecological physical therapists, and other health-care providers gives the client a well-rounded opportunity to heal and realize sexual health.

Why Ask about Sex?

Barratt and Rand give us three reasons why we should address sexuality routinely:[1]

1. Sexuality is part of who we are and the basis for functioning.
2. Because of the degree of cultural conflict, sexuality is a major struggle within an individual.
3. Due to internal and cultural conflict, sex is expressed in a risky fashion, so sexually transmitted disease and pregnancy are rampant.

Barratt and Rand suggest six "lines of questioning":

1. Sexual activity—how much sexual activity is there, and what gender are the partners?
2. Arousal—are there difficulties becoming or staying aroused?
3. Orgasmic satisfaction—are there difficulties reaching orgasm?
4. Medical considerations—are there medical issues that affect sexual pleasure?
5. General invitation—what other sexual concerns or questions are there?
6. Risk-reductive sexual counseling—what information about sexually-transmitted infections is known?

PLISSIT MODEL

A therapeutic model that is used to approach more difficult issues, such as sex, is the PLISSIT model.[2] The acronym is explained as follows:

- *Permission:* The therapist gives permission to the client by using a statement to help normalize the issue. The therapist, in order to provide a comfortable place to share difficult topics, fosters a safe environment. An example: "You've mentioned the relationship conflict. How has this affected sex with each other?"

- *Limited Information:* The therapist gives the client general information and corrects any misinformation. An example: "In talking about the rapid ejaculation that you're experiencing, let's keep in mind that there are many ways to sexually satisfy your partner even after you've ejaculated."
- *Specific Suggestion:* The therapist gives guidance to the client regarding interventions or particular ways to cope. An example: "How do you both feel about trying a sensate focus exercise to deal with the erectile difficulties? This is a type of caressing exercise that . . . "
- *Intensive Therapy:* The therapist moves on to a deeper level of therapy, if needed, focusing on other issues that might be contributing to the problem. Referrals will be made to other health-care providers, when necessary. An example: "It seems that we need to look into the bipolar issues that you've been diagnosed with and the effects of your medications on your sexual desire. I'd like to refer you to a urogynecological physiotherapist to help with the vaginal pain that you're having."

MOVING ACROSS THE BRIDGE

Sometimes you might find it necessary to seek help from others. In order to find the right person to help, you need to do a little background work. This saves you the time, money, and commitment that go into starting a therapeutic relationship that may not be the right one. Therapy can be scary, but it is also one of the most intimate (not in a sexual way!) relationships you will ever have in your life. Why not put some work into finding the therapist you can put your trust into in order to be able to reveal your sexual self?

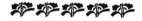

SEXERCISES

I. If you are considering therapy, think about what characteristics would be important to you in a therapist. Write these characteristics down.

Do some research on credible websites and in books about different types of therapists, different kinds of treatment, and different styles of therapy. Take notes about questions you may have for a therapist regarding therapy.

II. Research your particular problem and look at different ways it's being treated by therapists. Write down some questions for a therapist regarding the treatment of your issue and goals for therapy.

TALKING WITH YOUR
HEALTH-CARE PROVIDER

- Do you feel comfortable bringing up sex with your health-care provider?
- Does your health-care provider bring up the subject of sex?
- Does your health-care provider address sexual problems associated with illness or medication side effects?
- Are you a health-care provider who is having trouble discussing sexual issues with your patients?

With a new openness about sex among not only the younger generation, but also the baby boomers who lived through the sexual revolution, more adults of all ages are looking for a satisfying sex life. This new openness and desire for healthy sexuality brings with it the problems and disorders regarding sex, which need to be addressed by health-care providers. How does a person bring up sensitive problems like sex to their health-care provider?

THANKS, VIAGRA AND BOB DOLE!

Since Bob Dole "came out" about erectile dysfunction and Viagra appeared on the market, sexuality has been a topic we want more information about, and we want it from credible resources. As a species, we are living longer and having sex longer, but we need help! With age, stress, and life in general come little nuisances such as premature ejaculation, orgasmic difficulties, and vaginal dryness. In order to seek the best sex life we can have, we must open the lines of communication—not only with our partner, but also with our health-care provider.

It would be so much easier if all health-care providers were well versed in the area of sex and brought up the subject to their patients. It would be great if providers asked questions like "Have you noticed any sexual problems with this medication?" or "How is orgasmic satisfaction for you?" Unfortunately, not all health-care providers are taught about diagnosing sexual problems in medical school, and when you add to the equation the time constraints of managed health care, questions like this don't always get asked. As a society, we seem to learn more about sex from television or women's magazines than we do from the medical community, which means the information we receive is often sensationalized or incorrect. Our sexuality is such a big part of who we are, yet no one, except maybe our fifth-grade "health" teacher, gives us any facts about our sexual function. Seriously, how informative was that?! As adults, how many of us know very much about our sexual "parts"? What is a vulva? Where exactly is the perineum? What function does the prostate play? Where is the clitoris and how do I turn mine on?

Yvonne Fulbright states that some physicians don't provide this kind of information to their clients due to "bias, anxiety, gaps in knowledge, misconceptions, and discomfort with the subject."[1] Even though this might be understandable, it doesn't help the man with erectile dysfunction, the menopausal woman who is having problems with vaginal dryness, or the person who is uncomfortable with his or her gender and needs to discuss the matter with a health-care professional.

Anatomy and physiology aside, a patient needs to be able to ask frank questions about sexual health. It's up to the patient to find a health-care provider who can answer questions regarding sexual function. Even though it might be uncomfortable and difficult, sexual matters should be open for discussion in the examination room.

Wally and Wendy were just beginning their relationship and came to couples therapy telling the therapist that they were having difficulty with sex due to Wendy's genital pain. The therapist recommended that Wendy see her physician, in order to rule out any physical reasons she might be having pain. Wendy told the therapist that she tried to talk to her physician and was told to "go home, drink a glass of wine, and relax!" Wendy and Wally were left with the message that the problem was psychological. At this point, it very well might have been psychological, but medical reasons should always be ruled out when it comes to physical symptoms. The therapist suggested Wendy see a gynecologist, who specializes in women's sexual reproductive organs, before assuming the cause was psychological. Wendy and the therapist discussed different ways to address her issue with the new doctor so that she was able to get the help she needed. Because of the pain, Wendy was nervous about a pelvic exam, so the therapist taught her relaxation techniques in order to help her relax before the exam.

FINDING THE RIGHT HEALTH-CARE PROVIDER

There are different types of health-care providers that might be treating us at any given time. Let's take a look at different types of providers and what they do.

Physician (MD)

Physicians are medical doctors who spend four years in medical school and treat many different types of illness. Some physicians practice medicine in a general sense, while others choose specialties. A licensure process at the state level and certification through national organizations regulates the field of medicine.

Physician (DO)

Doctors of osteopathic medicine spend four years in medical school, and then receive extra instruction in the study of hands-on manual medicine and the body's musculoskeletal system. Osteopathic medicine seeks to treat and heal the patient as a whole. Osteopathic doctors can become specialized, with similar criteria as medical doctors.

Nurse Practitioner

A nurse practitioner is a nurse with a graduate degree in advanced practical nursing. Nurse practitioners can diagnose and treat disease, as well as prescribe medications and perform some procedures. Nurse practitioners may or may not be supervised by a physician, depending on the state in which they are practicing.

Physician's Assistant

The physician's assistant can provide health-care services with the direction and responsible supervision of a physician. Functions include diagnostic, therapeutic, preventive, and health maintenance services.

Internist

An internist is a physician who has completed a residency in internal medicine and practices long-term adult medicine.

Physical Therapist

Physical therapists return function, improve movement, relieve pain, and prevent or limit permanent disabilities of patients suffering from injuries or disease. Some physical therapists have advanced training in treating pelvic floor disorders. There is more on this specialty in appendix B, regarding women's genital pain disorders.

Urologist

A urologist is a doctor who specializes in the male reproductive urological system.

Gynecologist

A gynecologist is a doctor who specializes in the care of women and their reproductive organs.

HOW DO I TALK TO MY HEALTH-CARE PROVIDER ABOUT SEX?

Now that we have more information about health-care providers, it's time to discuss how to broach the subject of sex. As we discussed earlier, due to managed care, health-care providers have very little time in the examination room. It's up to us to tell the provider what our concerns are and ask appropriate questions, because, chances are, the provider won't have time to address every aspect of our bodies. It's important to keep in mind that providers don't have a crystal ball, so if we are having sexual problems, we have to say so when we have their attention. What are examples of good questions for our providers?

- Will there be any sexual side effects with that medication or treatment?
- Is it normal that sex has become less frequent because of _____?
- Is there a way we can enhance sexual arousal?
- Do you know of a good sex therapist who can help me?
- Is pain in the vaginal area normal during sex?
- Is there anything I can do to slow down ejaculation during intercourse?
- What do you suggest regarding my lack of erections?

Finding an Understanding Provider

If you feel more comfortable talking with a particular gender, seek that gender out in your health-care provider. It might be worth it to bring up sexual concerns when making the appointment. As mental health providers, we appreciate it when someone gives a brief idea of what the presenting problem is on the phone. We can save the person time and money by steering them in the right direction, if needed. Check the website www.aasect.org if a sex therapist might be helpful. Ask friends and family to recommend someone they have seen for a similar problem.

Before the first appointment, many people find it helpful to write down questions they want answered. Research your particular problem so that you have a fairly good idea of what you need to know. Be prepared! Patients need to walk away from the provider's office feeling as though their questions were answered in a respectful manner. When we have trouble talking about a sexual issue, we can try bringing in an article or brochure to help break the ice on the topic.

Keep in mind that if the health-care provider doesn't seem to have the expertise to help or isn't listening to concerns, every patient has the right to ask for a referral to a specialist who is an expert in that area.

🌿 SEXUAL HEALING

I am so embarrassed! I did all my homework and wrote down questions for my health-care provider, and guess what?! It's like he didn't even hear me! Low desire is really hurting my relationship, and I'm so disappointed . . . I thought this would help. I'm feeling unheard and like there's no hope. . . . If I can't count on my doctor to help, am I doomed to a crappy sex life?

Don't give up! It sounds like you did your part. Assuming that you clearly expressed your problem, it's not your fault that the provider wasn't able to hear you. Providers are human, and have their own biases and feelings about sex. If this provider didn't help you, look elsewhere. It's difficult to put yourself out there and be vulnerable, only to walk away feeling unheard. Don't stop there. Ask around, make phone calls, and find a provider who will be sensitive to your needs.

🌿 🌿 🌿

DO I REALLY HAVE TO GO THERE?

If you are a health-care provider and have difficulty talking about sexual issues with your patients, it's important to figure out what makes "the sex talk" difficult for you. We all have our issues, but sex is as important to a person as their cardiovascular system or the condition of their skin. When it comes to happiness and relationship satisfaction, our sex life can play a huge part, not to mention the great health benefits of satisfying sexual encounters.

As we've emphasized throughout this book, it might be useful to think about your childhood messages about sex. Was shame prevalent when you were growing up? What are your own reactions to sex, as an adult? All these factors play in to how we talk about sex with our partners, patients, or our own health-care providers. Sometimes it's helpful to involve other types of practitioners, making up an interdisciplinary team to help the patient with sexual concerns. There are great sex therapists and physical therapists who are well-trained in the area of sex. www. aasect.org is a good resource to find sex therapists so that providers can refer their patients for this specialty. There's even a map on the website so that you and your patient can find someone in your geographic area.

How Do I Bring It Up?

It's important to remember that not every patient is heterosexual. Try not to assume, as they may have difficulty bringing up the topic of orientation or transgender issues. Health-care providers can follow many models when considering how to discuss sex with their patients. One is the BETTER model, which suggests touching on the following:[2]

- Bring the topic up, giving permission to talk about sexual concerns.
- Explain that sex is a part of life, therefore normalizing the patient's concerns.
- Tell patients that there are resources and perhaps provide them with websites and a resource list.
- Time the intervention correctly, making sure the timing is appropriate.
- Educate about side effects of treatment.
- Record (to remember to revisit the issue).

As a health-care provider, you don't have the ability to know everything the patient is dealing with, but bringing up the topic of sex can help a patient know that it's safe to present those issues in the examining room. Addressing the issue of sex can be as simple as asking a question such as, "Do you have any sexual concerns today?" or, "Are you practicing safe sex?" It gives permission to talk about sex when the patient feels the need.

MOVING ACROSS THE BRIDGE

When sexual difficulty is occurring, who better to consider talking to than your health-care provider (besides your partner, of course)? There are interventions that can help and the problem might be solved by a change in medication or another treatment approach. Find a health-care provider with whom you can feel comfortable and who will point you in the right direction if the issue is beyond his or her own expertise. Most importantly, don't give up if you have a disappointing experience. Be proactive in finding the help you need.

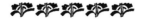

SEXERCISES

I. If you have a particular physical problem, do your homework and research the problem. Seek out Internet information, books, and pamphlets that might be helpful to you. Make a list of questions to ask your health-care provider.

II. Are you taking a specific medication or treatment? Get as much information as you can about that treatment, then write down questions for your health-care provider about any sexual concerns.

III. Write down any sexual concerns you might have for your provider. If you have information about that concern, take it with you to an appointment so that you can show the provider what you have learned.

APPENDICES

Ⓐ

MALE SEXUAL DISORDERS

This section will describe common male sexual disorders and helpful tools for dealing with each disorder. Sexual difficulties may result from lack of sexual education, illness or disability, use of medication, the aging process, situational factors, substance use or abuse, relationship concerns, psychological and emotional issues, and any combination of the above. It's important to remember that any sexual performance or pleasure issue needs to be viewed from a biopsychosocial perspective; in other words, keep in mind the physical, emotional, and relational contributors to any problem that you are experiencing.

This appendix is a brief guide to the most common male sexual disorders and is not meant to be exhaustive in description or in treatment options. Please keep in mind that it is important to discuss your sexual issues with both your partner and your health-care provider. You may also find it helpful to explore your sexual needs and difficulties with a therapist. Chapters 10 and 11 give tips on ways to bring up these topics to your therapist or health-care provider. Included in the resources section of this book are books, videos, and websites that can help in the understanding and treatment of the following sexual disorders.

As you explore the following sexual issues for men, please keep in mind that there are several important factors to consider. First, you need to determine if this sexual concern is causing *you* distress or if it is causing your partner distress. If the sexual issue does not distress you, you may be satisfied to leave things well enough alone. However, if you feel that the sexual concern is a couple's issue, you may need to discuss this with your partner, and a therapist or physician. Second, in exploring the sexual issue, you need to determine if it occurs situationally (only with one partner and not another, or only at certain times and not others) or if it occurs generally (in all circumstances). Third, investigate whether the sexual concern is lifelong (primary) or acquired (secondary). Has this disorder been with you your entire life, as long as you can remember, or did it develop only after some event or situation? Looking at these factors can help you describe your situation to your partner, health-care provider, or therapist.

RAPID EJACULATION

Rapid ejaculation, formerly called premature ejaculation, is one of the most common sexual problems reported by men. However, it's somewhat difficult to define rapid ejaculation because sometimes a man, or his partner, will complain of early ejaculation based on a subjective measure that the couple or individual has determined qualifies for *too soon*. With rapid ejaculation, the man feels he is not in control of his experience and will ejaculate either right before intromission, during intromission, or within seconds or a minute or two of thrusting.

It's important to note that the typical sexual encounter for most couples lasts about 15 to 45 minutes and includes 2 to 7 minutes of intercourse.[1] It may be surprising that the actual intercourse experience isn't a marathon event, given media myths or folklore. Men and couples are vulnerable to the hype suggesting that *good* sexual intercourse lasts a long time and is always satisfying for both partners.

Some men with rapid ejaculation will attempt to slow down their sexual response with the use of desensitizing creams or by thinking of distracting or negative thoughts. However, this isn't an effective method to slow down ejaculation and only reduces arousal. It's common that a man will experience rapid ejaculation as dissatisfying and embarrassing and may have difficulty talking about this disorder with his partner or physician.

There are many possible causes for rapid ejaculation. For some men, there might be a genetic predisposition such that the sympathetic nervous system is overly sensitive, leading to a quick reflex in the pelvic muscles. Physical illness, such as urinary tract infection or prostate infection, may affect ejaculatory speed. At times, the use or discontinuation of a medication or drug can lead to rapid ejaculation. It's necessary, then, to explore this issue with your physician, especially if it's a recent occurrence.

There are many psychological contributors, both individual and within the relationship, which affect ejaculation. The man may feel anxiety, depression, anger, restrictive beliefs, lack of confidence, and so on. The couple may be struggling with relationship conflict, fears, disappointments, and even the partner's sexual concerns (inhibited desire, anxiety, sexual negativity, etc.). Finally, a man may lack accurate information about his body, his partner's body, sexuality skills or techniques, or realistic expectations about sexuality and performance.

Metz and McCarthy point out that learning ejaculatory control involves identifying the point of ejaculatory inevitability.[2] This is the point at which ejaculation is no longer a voluntary function and the man will ejaculate, no matter what. Ejaculatory control also involves increasing comfort, physical and emotional awareness, and stimulation. It can be helpful for a man struggling with rapid ejaculation to practice his arousal and response while masturbating, either alone or with his partner present. During masturbation, the man can learn what techniques might be helpful to slow down his arousal.

A man can learn better control through self-stimulation; however, eventually the learning and practice will need to be incorporated into the sexual interaction with his partner. There may be difficulty when transitioning from self-understanding and solitary practice to sexual intercourse. It'll require that the couple be open in their communication and that they share realistic performance goals. It's a good idea for a couple to explore the diagnosis and treatment of rapid ejaculation together, through reading or viewing an educational video (you can find one at the Sinclair Institute website, included in the resources section of this book). If a man and his partner are having a great deal of relationship conflict, either about the rapid ejaculation or about some other matter, it will be difficult to proceed with a team approach. Sometimes it becomes necessary for the couple to seek counseling to relieve or lessen the emotional conflict before proceeding to intercourse.

Arousal can be viewed on a 10-point scale, with "0" being neutral and "10" being orgasm. On this scale, "5" is the beginning of erection and "8" is high arousal sensations. Metz and McCarthy encourage the male with rapid ejaculation to become keenly aware of his arousal according to this scale.[3] Once he has become tuned into his unique arousal pattern, he then learns to move from "5" to "10" very slowly with attention to his own personal sensations rather than giving too much attention, initially, to partner interaction. Using the "stop-start" technique, the man, and then the couple, learns to stop stimulation as the man approaches ejaculatory inevitability. Stimulation stops for a few seconds, until the man no longer feels the need to ejaculate, and then stimulation resumes. This takes a great deal of practice and patience. It *is* possible to achieve better ejaculatory control. It's advisable for the man to practice using self-stimulation until he reaches an adequate level of self-understanding and can then progress to sexual activity with his partner.

For a couple, rapid ejaculation can be a very challenging and complex problem with which to deal. It requires patience, empathetic listening, and cooperation to move from a problematic sexual encounter to one that is enjoyable and satisfying. However, with practice and exploration, it can be accomplished. When moving from self-stimulation to intercourse, it's usually better to use the woman-on-top position, as this provides more control for the man. At first, it's advisable to engage in intercourse with little or no movement. Movement can be introduced slowly as the man gains control and comfort with his partner's interaction and stimulation. The man can stimulate his partner in ways other than intercourse so that the partner can experience pleasure and satisfaction. Recall that, for many women, intercourse alone will not lead to orgasm; therefore, ejaculatory control (and prolonged intercourse thrusting) is not necessary for a woman to experience pleasure and/or orgasm. Likewise, a woman may not feel that she needs an orgasm in order to feel sexual and emotional fulfillment.

In some situations, the use of an antidepressant medication is prescribed along with the other techniques described above. A low dose of a selective serotonin reuptake inhibitor (such as Paxil or Celexa) will often promote ejaculatory control; however, the success of this regimen is dependent upon remaining on the medication, unless the "stop-start" technique is incorporated. A man may be able to use the medication for a while, eventually lower the dose, gradually implement the "stop-start" technique, and then reduce or eliminate the pharmacologic intervention. Focus on the awareness of pleasure and don't allow the fear of rapid ejaculation to interfere with arousal.

ERECTILE DISORDER

It's normal that, by age forty, most males experience at least one erectile failure. This doesn't mean that an erectile disorder should be diagnosed at this time or that the erectile failure will necessarily occur often. Erectile disorder is defined as the inability to achieve or maintain an erection sufficient for sexual performance. Erectile dysfunction is more prevalent in aging men, affecting approximately half of all men older than sixty.[4] The incidence of erectile dysfunction is correlated with risk factors, such as cardiovascular disease, diabetes, depression, and lower urinary tract symptoms. An unhealthy lifestyle, such as smoking, lack of exercise, obesity, and alcohol abuse, is also a predictor of erectile dysfunction. Additionally, fatigue, hormonal deficiency, and side effects of medication are all possible contributors to erectile failure. A thorough medical exam is necessary, as erectile dysfunction may be an early marker for cardiovascular and other disease states. A physician can also help a man consider his lifestyle, hormone levels, and medication interactions to determine the appropriate treatment for the disorder, deficiency, or medical concern.

The widespread use of Viagra and other "pro-erection" oral medications (PDE5 inhibitors) has revolutionized sexual dysfunction in men. These medications appear to be effective in restoring erections for about 75 percent of men who use them.[5] However, many men are never assessed by their physician for psychological contributors for erectile failure, but are instead prescribed one of the three pro-erection aids (Viagra, Cialis, and Levitra). In fact, there may be psychological or interpersonal issues that are affecting the man with erectile failure, such as lack of sexual desire, relationship conflict, rapid ejaculation, or delayed/inhibited ejaculation.

A substantial proportion of men with erectile dysfunction discontinue the use of the oral medications. In a recent study of more than 25,000 men in eight countries, it was determined that 58 percent of men with erection problems had discussed the problem with their physician, fewer than half of these men received a pro-erection prescription, and only 16 percent were continuing to use the drug at the time of the study.[6] The discontinuation may be due to the fear of side effects, partner concerns, distrust of medications, failed expectations, lack of education regarding the medication, or a lack of change in the quality of the sexual relationship.

There are several possible psychological determinants of erectile failure. Problems such as lack of adequate stimulation, lack of understanding regarding the normal aging process, performance anxiety or fear of failure, and relationship conflicts (communication difficulties, lack of intimacy or trust, and power conflicts) may all take their toll on the male and his ability to get and maintain an erection. Past experiences may also play a role in erectile failure, such as sexual trauma, sexual identity issues, unresolved parental attachments, and cultural or religious taboos.

One of the fundamental keys to understanding and treating erectile failure is in the psychosexual development of males. Young men learn, during puberty, that their sexual response is predictable, automatic, and autonomous. A teenage boy will usually experience easy erections and can have arousal and orgasm without the interaction of a partner. This early learning, however, does not translate well for men as they age or are in long-term relationships. Because the neurological, vascular, and hormonal systems are functioning at their prime in the early years, erectile function is usually predictable and reliable. As men age, their vascular and neurological functioning is less efficient; therefore, the psychological and interpersonal aspects of the sexual encounter cannot be ignored or taken for granted.

After medical, lifestyle, and hormonal concerns have been addressed, a couple will need to practice patience and explore options for sensual enhancement. It's important for the individual not to fall into the trap of believing that he is always going to be ready and able to keep a firm erection for an entire lovemaking session. In a forty-five-minute sexual encounter, an erection will wax and wane two to five times, and this process is not an indication of lack of desire.[7] It's critical not to label erectile changes as a definitive diagnosis of impotence because many of these changes are temporary and situation-specific. Erectile problems don't affect the ability to ejaculate, as a man can ejaculate with a flaccid penis.

Most men realize that it's not possible to force or *will* an erection. However, it's easy to forget that an erect penis is actually not necessary for partner satisfaction. A partner can experience orgasm through many avenues of stimulation or may enjoy the comfort and pleasure of touch without orgasm.

It's helpful for a man to practice different types of stimulation during masturbation so that he can increase his understanding of his own arousal pattern. This self-knowledge can be shared with his partner, verbally or nonverbally. It may be necessary to directly show or verbally express the specific movement and speed needed, as many men require increased stimulation, especially as they age. Not all sexual encounters are satisfying, and it's not unusual to have setbacks or even failures. Recall the good-enough sex model, described in chapter 7, as this encourages couples to enjoy the pleasure and intimacy of their sexual relationship without being overly frustrated by the inevitable variability of sexual functioning.[8]

At times, a man and his physician may determine that a trial on a pro-erection aid is advisable. These aids may be in the form of oral medication or another device (such as intracavernous drugs by injection to the penis, a suppository into the urethra containing medication, or a vacuum constriction device). To increase the likelihood of success using the erectile aid, it's best to integrate the medical intervention into a lovemaking style that is interactive, patient, sensual, and fun. Practicing pelvic floor strengthening exercises may help some men regain erectile control and improved erections. There is a sexercise on Kegels in chapter 9 explaining how to strengthen the pelvic floor muscles.

It can be helpful for a couple to implement sensate focus exercises in order to remove the pressure to perform. The exercises can be simply an exploration of arousal. The couple might determine that orgasm and intercourse are not the objective at this time and just enjoy touching for the sake of touching. Sensate focus exercises are helpful to allow for exploration and pleasure without the anxiety that often becomes associated with erectile performance. Appendix C contains more information on sensate focus exercises.

LOW DESIRE

Men often find it difficult to talk about a lowering of sexual desire. Unfortunately, in our culture, it's assumed that females suffer from low desire, but that males are sexual machines. However, inhibited sexual desire is more common for men than many people believe. The prime source of population-based information, the National Health and Social Life Survey interviews, found that 16 percent of men reported they had experienced lack of interest in sex, lasting several months, during the past twelve months.[9] In some relationships, the male makes the decision to avoid sexual intercourse. This can be a surprising fact for some, but it appears that when men feel that intercourse is not an option—for one reason or another—they back away, usually nonverbally, from sexual interaction and other forms of intimacy and affection. There are several possible contributors to lowered sexual desire in men.

Recall that most males and females are under the impression that men *always* want sex and are *always* able to perform on demand. As discussed in earlier sections of this book, performance is not something that men can reliably count on every time. With age, medication usage, stress, fatigue, hormone imbalances, and illness, erections are not always dependable. Once erection concerns develop, a man may find that he feels discouraged or embarrassed and backs away from sexual encounters. He may still feel some sexual desire, but it can easily develop into a confusing cycle of disappointment and fear leading to avoidance. The struggle with self-confidence then often leads to a lowering of desire.

There are many psychological contributors to low desire. At times, the relationship is stressed and conflict is either overt or simmering under the surface. When relationship discord continues for a long period or a man feels excessively criticized or rejected (direct rejection or even perceived rejection), his desire and/or confidence may diminish. At times, it's difficult for a man to feel comfortable with psychological intimacy and so he withdraws from the closeness required to engage in sexual activity and arousal. Men who are depressed or highly anxious may also find that sexual intercourse is not highly desired. A man's low desire can be entangled in his partner's low desire or another sexual disorder, such as anorgasmia or pain with intercourse. At times, a man can become dependent upon a certain type of arousal (such as a paraphilia or pornographic material), and subsequently find it difficult to become involved with someone in an intimate relationship or to become aroused by something other than the specific desired stimulus.

The physical issues that might lead to low desire—hormone imbalances, medication side effects, and illness—should be explored with a physician. Biological contributors will need to be ruled out before psychological contributors can be examined. It may be that the physical, psychological, and relational factors combine to create diminished sexual desire. If a man is prescribed an antidepressant for clinical depression and the medication results in an erectile disorder, he may find that he withdraws from his partner sexually. The cycle of depression, medication side effects, erectile failure, and relationship challenges can easily lead to low desire. Men sometimes report that "it's just not worth it." The partner of a man with low desire will need to be encouraging and understanding in order to explore the factors that may be influencing the diminished desire.

In some cases, a man will need to discuss his lowered sexual desire with a therapist in order to explore all of the factors and causes that may be contributing to his problem. A couple needs to be encouraged to discuss any potential issues that might be leading to relationship distress. For a man, it's likely challenging to talk about low desire because this is a concept that males have difficulty accepting in our culture. However, it is much better to talk openly about the changes in desire than allow the subject to drain the relationship. Often a female will talk, in therapy, about her partner's low desire as "the elephant in the room."

Being able to explore the following questions may be helpful:

- What makes sex appealing?
- What has put me in the mood in the past?
- In what situations do I feel sexual desire?
- What turns me off?
- What was happening in my life when my libido was higher than it is now?
- When I do feel desire, what do I usually do with that feeling (ignore it, act on it, feel shame, distract myself)?
- What are sensory triggers that turn me on?
- When my partner acts sexually interested, how do I interpret this?

Being open to enjoy affectionate interaction and intimacy without the pressure to perform is the key to a revitalized sexual relationship. When it comes to sexual activity, using a sensate focus approach or caressing activity will also enhance the ability to remain connected and explore sexual turn-ons.

DELAYED EJACULATION

Delayed or inhibited ejaculation is the inability to be orgasmic despite being physically aroused and erect. There are different manifestations of delayed ejaculation. Most males with delayed ejaculation report that they are able to orgasm during masturbation, but not during intercourse. Some also are unable to orgasm with partner oral or manual stimulation. This may be an intermittent problem or a chronic difficulty. It might occur with some partners, but not with all partners.

Men do not report this disorder as often as they report rapid ejaculation or erectile disorder, but it *is* found in males, especially over the age of fifty. Prevalence rates are difficult to determine, as the dysfunction may be misdiagnosed as an erection or desire problem. The most common form of ejaculatory inhibition is coital anorgasmia, in which the man is able to achieve orgasm through manual or oral stimulation, but not through intercourse.

The possible causes of ejaculatory inhibition are many. Depression, side effects of medications, fatigue, anxiety, excessive masturbation, alcohol or drug abuse, and the inability to request certain sexual preferences are some of the likely reasons. Many times, the struggle with ejaculatory inhibition will lead to low sexual desire, the avoidance of sex and even of all types of touch, and finally to a nonsexual relationship.

A common cause for ejaculatory inhibition is that the couple has fallen into a routine of intercourse that is mechanical. When a man transitions to intercourse at the start of his erection, he may not be at a high-enough level of arousal to achieve orgasm, especially with a partner. This will lead to frustration and possibly the loss of erection.

Perelman and Rowland, in writing about delayed ejaculation, explains that one reason men can have difficulty reaching orgasm with a partner might be masturbatory practices that don't transfer well to intercourse.[10]

He encourages men with this disorder to think of masturbation as a "dress rehearsal" for sex with one's partner. He elaborates that the couple can view the delayed ejaculatory struggle as simply that the man is unprepared for his particular part in the play. The author suggests that the man use fantasy and bodily movements during intercourse that are similar to the sensations (pressure, speed, and technique) and thoughts that he has experienced with masturbation.

It's important that couples talk about the type of stimulation that they each personally require in order to achieve necessary levels of arousal. Transitioning to intercourse when the arousal level is high, not at the start of an erection, will help to maintain the intensity of stimulation needed. Although a man may have objective evidence that he is aroused, such as a firm erection, he may not be sufficiently aroused internally or psychologically.

The couple should find ways to incorporate various types of stimulation that they both find arousing. It may be tempting to assume that the type of erotic sensuality employed in the early relationship or in youth continues to be effective. However, it's helpful to explore whether gentle sexual activity or a more interactive and active style is preferred, as turn-ons change with time. Explore what orgasm triggers may exist (such as certain places to be touched or caressed, different positions, specific types of movement or speeds of movement, tensing pelvic muscles, and verbalizing arousal). It's understandable, given our culture's assumption about male performance, that a discussion about delayed ejaculation will be uncomfortable for many couples. However, it's necessary to talk about the possible causes of the disorder and the usefulness of experimentation with new sexual stimulation techniques.

SENSATE FOCUS

We have mentioned the helpfulness of using sensate focus with the above sexual disorders. Sensate focus is sensual massage or comforting touch that is not meant to necessarily include orgasm or intercourse. Appendix C contains helpful information about sensate focus; we encourage you and your partner to read it and talk about trying some of the exercises.

(B)

FEMALE SEXUAL DISORDERS

This section will describe common female sexual disorders and helpful tools for dealing with each disorder. Sexual difficulties may result from lack of sexual education, illness or disability, use of medication, the aging process, situational factors, substance use or abuse, relationship concerns, psychological and emotional issues, and any combination of the above. It's important to remember that any sexual performance or pleasure issue needs to be viewed from a biopsychosocial perspective; in other words, keep in mind the physical, emotional, and relational contributors to any problem that you are experiencing.

This appendix is a brief guide to the most common female sexual disorders and is not meant to be exhaustive in description or in treatment options. Please keep in mind that it is important to discuss your sexual issues with both your partner and your health-care provider. You may also find it helpful to explore your sexual needs and difficulties with a therapist. Chapters 10 and 11 give tips on ways to bring up these topics with your therapist or health-care provider. Included in the recommended resources section of this book are books, videos, and websites that can help in the understanding and treatment of these sexual disorders.

As you explore the following sexual issues for women, please keep in mind that there are several important factors to consider. First, you need to determine if this sexual concern is causing *you* distress or if it is causing your partner distress. If the sexual issue does not distress you, you may be satisfied to leave things well enough alone. However, if you feel that the sexual concern is a couple's issue, you may need to discuss this with your partner, and a therapist or physician. Second, in exploring the sexual issue, you need to determine if it occurs situationally (only with one partner and not another, or only at certain times and not others) or if it occurs generally (in all circumstances). Third, investigate whether the sexual concern is lifelong (primary) or acquired (secondary). Has this disorder been with you your entire life, as long as you can remember, or did it develop only after some event or situation? Looking at these factors can help you describe your situation to your partner, health-care provider, or therapist.

LOW DESIRE

Low libido is found among women of all ages and is one of the most common sexual complaints among women and their partners. Sexual desire is influenced by many different factors such as culture, upbringing, sexual education/knowledge, body image, self-esteem, relationship difficulties, communication with partner, emotional issues (such as depression or anxiety), medications and herbs, medical procedures, hormonal imbalances, and so on.

Low desire doesn't have to lead to total avoidance of sexual intimacy or obligatory dysfunctional sex. Because so many things can influence sexual desire, it's important to view desire issues with an open and investigative mind. Lack of desire is complex and the sources are very individual. Avoid blame and instead work together to find ways to enrich the sexual relationship. If there is a medication that's contributing to lowered desire, a physician may be able to choose another medication. Hormone levels may need to be evaluated.

The psychological contributors to low desire in women should be explored, as well. Sometimes unresolved conflict is poisoning a relationship, so address these issues either on your own or with the help of a trained therapist. Many women describe being fatigued and having little time for themselves. This necessitates a discussion about how to set aside time to relax and/or organize help with chores and errands. The relationship needs to be examined, as so often women describe feeling disconnected from their partner.

For some women, especially those who are older or in long-term relationships, there might not be a strong instinctive drive for sexual pleasure. These women find that their sexual response cycle begins in a neutral state rather than with an intense awareness of sexual desire.[1] However, if a woman chooses, she can consider nonsexual and emotional motivators (such as desiring closeness, connection, and bonding), which may lead her to seek sexual stimulation. When a woman chooses sexual stimulation, it often leads to physical arousal. Physical arousal, in turn, leads to an awareness of the desire to continue stimulation for sexual and nonsexual reasons. Arousal and desire may or may not progress to orgasm for the woman. Even without orgasm, the woman can still experience a full sense of emotional and physical satisfaction. This model is circular rather than linear: the woman's physical and emotional response loops back to the emotional motivators that will likely lead her to desire sexual interaction at other times. The Basson model is described in more detail in chapter 4.

For many women, sexual desire is not automatic but can be elicited by emotional and relational factors with her partner. It's helpful to know what factors contribute to desire for a sexual relationship. These contributors to desire will likely change somewhat over a woman's lifetime.

Explore the following questions:

- What makes sex appealing?
- What's put me in the mood in the past?
- In what situations do I feel sexual desire?
- What turns me off?
- What was happening in my life when my libido was higher than it is now?
- When I do feel desire, what do I usually do with that feeling (ignore it, act on it, feel shame, distract myself)?
- What are sensory triggers that turn me on?
- When my partner acts sexually interested, how do I interpret this?

It's important to be open to exploring your own desire and arousal in order to enhance and rekindle your sexual relationship. Using sensate focus exercises or sensual massage can lead to a reconnection to your sexual self and to your partner. Appendix C contains more information regarding sensate focus exercises.

LACK OF SEXUAL AROUSAL

Female arousal includes blood flow to the clitoris, vaginal lubrication, the expansion of the upper part of the vagina, uterus, cervix and clitoris, and the swelling of the lower labia and vagina. However, many things can inhibit arousal, and women sometimes explain that they feel physically and emotionally numb when it comes to libido. Similar things that lower sexual desire also lower arousal: hormonal changes, stress, relationship problems, medical procedures, medications, ineffective sexual techniques or stimulation, and so on.

A water-based lubricant before and during sexual play can help with sexual arousal. Lubrication allows for more extended playtime, which can lead to increased stimulation and excitement. If there's vaginal dryness resulting from a decrease in estrogen, a physician might prescribe hormone replacement therapy or estrogen applied directly to the vulva area, which helps the vaginal tissue to remain rejuvenated and moist. Examining the emotional issues in the relationship can help alleviate some of the stressors that can be distracting from sexual arousal. Finally, allowing for exploration of eroticism can stimulate the imagination and the body. Arousal is stirred by the mind and at times the imagination needs to be awakened. We have included books and websites about erotica in the resources section. Reading something sexy or watching a video that portrays stimulating erotic scenes may inspire you and your partner.

ORGASMIC DISORDER

The ability to experience orgasm is influenced by mood, hormonal changes, fatigue, lack of sexual knowledge or experimentation, inhibitions, many biological issues (such as medications, illnesses, etc.), relationship factors (such as conflict or power struggles), and so on. What if medication is absolutely necessary, say for depression, but the medication interferes greatly with desire, arousal, or orgasm? In these cases, talking about the medication with your physician might lead to choosing a medication that doesn't carry negative side effects. There are continuing studies being undertaken to determine if the use of Viagra can help with decreased sensitivity and absent or delayed orgasm in women who are taking antidepressants.[2] It appears that there may be some positive effects from the addition of Viagra for women taking selective serotonin reuptake inhibitors (SSRIs) such as Prozac, Paxil, Zoloft, and others. One study found that Viagra helped the women reach orgasm and improved their orgasm satisfaction. Other aspects, such as arousal, desire, and natural lubrication, improved less. This study regarding Viagra and SSRIs in women is ongoing and it will be interesting to see the findings of this, and other, investigations.

Arousal and orgasm can be challenging to achieve. Women don't need to reach orgasm with every sexual encounter in order for the experience to be enjoyable. Sexual play can be very erotic and stimulating, but not include orgasm, and the woman may still feel very satisfied and connected to her partner.

Many women are not able to achieve orgasm without direct clitoral stimulation. This is very normal. This means that the physical thrusting of the penis does not stimulate a woman in the most effective way to lead to orgasm. The clitoris might be directly stimulated by varying positions, self-stimulation, manual or oral stimulation by her partner, the use of a vibrator, and so on.

How do you go about making orgasm achievable? It can be a double-edged sword. Make it a priority, but don't become overly anxious about it at the same time. Here are some pointers:

- Take time to explore your body and know how you respond to different types of touch.
- Examine your genitals with a mirror and locate your clitoris, labia, and vaginal opening.
- Read about programs that help you achieve orgasm.
- Try not to be too goal-oriented. When you become anxious about your sexual experience, it's likely that your body will respond by constricting the blood vessels, diminishing arousal.
- Make sure that you can communicate your needs to your partner.

- Use lubrication, as it will help with dryness and aid in sensation.
- If you are comfortable using a vibrator, try it for stimulation and foreplay.
- Pay attention to what you feel you need in your environment— what to wear, what scents you might find relaxing or romantic, what music you might want to have on in the background, etc.
- Determine how stressed out you might be and whether this could interfere with your arousal. Take a bubble bath, perhaps, or delay sex until you feel more relaxed.
- If you are self-conscious about foreplay that is directed only at you, share in the foreplay. Mutuality may facilitate arousal and excitement.
- As you become more aware of what you need in order to feel aroused, guide your partner's hand or body or tell him or her verbally.
- Remember that orgasm can occur during foreplay, intercourse, or afterplay.
- It's unrealistic to expect orgasm during every sexual encounter. Sexuality is not about proving anything to yourself or your partner.
- Sometimes orgasm with a partner is much more challenging than with masturbation. And it can be difficult to transfer your knowledge about masturbatory orgasm to orgasm in partner sex. Chapter 7 has a sexercise that gives tips on how to do this.
- Appendix C has more information about sensate focus exercises that can help you explore arousal and orgasm.

GENITAL PAIN DISORDERS

The medical term for recurrent or persistent genital pain associated with sexual intercourse is dyspareunia. Dyspareunia can develop as a result of many different medical problems, such as thinning of the vaginal lining during menopause, vaginal infections, pain following vaginal and vulvar surgical procedures, endometriosis, injury, surgical nerve damage or scarring, tumors or cysts, interstitial cystitis, and many other conditions. Dyspareunia may also be emotionally based or reflect a relationship problem or conflict. The emotional component might also include past trauma or somatization of anger or anxiety. Sometimes dyspareunia is caused by a combination of biological, psychological, and relational factors.

There are physical conditions related to sexual pain that only a trained physician can diagnose and treat. For instance, some women may believe that they are suffering from yeast infections because they are experiencing a burning sensation around their genitals. However, the burning and irritation need to be examined and diagnosed by a health professional. A painful, burning rawness and inflammation might be due to localized provoked vulvodynia (the term used for vulvar pain), and a woman should be examined by her physician and follow the recommendations for treatment. The causes of localized provoked vulvodynia are not well understood. Cases of vulvodynia can be linked to hormone imbalances associated with oral contraceptives or the natural changes of hormones with aging. Additionally, there is evidence that, at times, the pain is associated with the firing of nerve bundles in the vulvar area.

Localized provoked vulvodynia is often a difficult condition to treat, but there is currently more research being done and physicians are able to help. Some of the possible treatments are oral medications, topical steroids, a low-oxalate diet, surgical removal of the affected area, or topical applications of anti-inflammatory compounded creams. Additionally, when women experience pain or a burning sensation that is due to dermatologic disorders, such as lichen sclerosus, a physician needs to be involved in the treatment of this disorder.

When a woman isn't fully aroused or lubricated, penetration can be uncomfortable. The use of added lubrication is not only recommended for those who are entering menopause, but also for women at any age—it can be useful to enhance arousal and lead to penetration that's more comfortable.

Another condition seen by physical and mental health providers is vaginismus. Vaginismus has been described as involuntary muscle spasms of the lower third of the vagina (almost like a blink; involuntary and reactive to real or anticipated pain). Because it's difficult to examine a woman with vaginismus, it's hard to determine if there are actual spasms taking place. Nevertheless, the anticipatory anxiety and tension interfere with penetration by the partner, and also may preclude the use of tampons and interfere with pelvic exams by a physician. Vaginismus usually develops as a conditioned response to the experience of painful penetration; however, it can be the result of relationship and emotional problems. Sometimes vaginismus involves a strong fear response based on past penetration trauma, past pain with intercourse, past medical procedures, or the belief that pain is likely to occur. At times, the emotional issues might be related to strict moral or religious ideology interfering with healthy sexual development and expression.

With dyspareunia, consultation for psychotherapy may be needed. When relationship conflict has become intense and painful intercourse is linked to anger and resentment, it's necessary to address the interpersonal issues. If sex has become obligatory, a woman may move to intercourse without being sufficiently aroused. The lack of arousal and lubrication will contribute to discomfort with penetration and this, in turn, will lead to the subsequent association of the pain response with intercourse. Exploring the emotional factors that may be barriers to intimacy can lead to increased desire and the pleasurable anticipation of intercourse.

Dyspareunia is best treated by the involvement of the partner, the physician, a sex therapist, and a specially trained urogynecological physical therapist. Urogynecological physiotherapists specialize in the treatment of sexual pain disorders. These specialists can offer anatomical and physiological education, cognitive-behavioral interventions, instruction in the use of vaginal dilators, biofeedback, advice for pelvic floor muscle strengthening, and relaxation exercises. When the pain is severe and not responsive to talking in therapy, it is important to seek the expertise of the physical therapist.

The urogynecological physiotherapist will conduct a thorough and private assessment, including a medical and sexual history, musculoskeletal examination, and vulvar and pelvic floor examination. Physical therapy includes the use of pelvic floor biofeedback, trigger point and connective tissue massage, instruction regarding Kegel exercises (to strengthen the pubococcygeus muscle), in-home use of dilators, deep breathing, relaxation, self-touch, desensitization, sensate focus, and much more. Intercourse positions which could lead to less discomfort or increased arousal are discussed. While a woman is seeing a physiotherapist for sexual pain, intercourse will likely not be possible at that time. However, affectionate touching needs to continue to occur and possibly some creative styles of intercourse, such as "outercourse," wherein thrusting of the penis is accomplished outside of the vagina, using the legs or breasts for friction.

Genital pain is a complex phenomenon and needs to be carefully assessed by a trained health-care professional. This treatment area is growing and developing constantly. New treatment protocols are regularly being explored and implemented. Treatment might require in-depth psychotherapy, medical intervention, and/or physical therapy. Keep in mind that genital pain is a treatable condition and is best viewed as a couple's issue since it's helpful to have the partner involved. The following is an excellent and frequently updated website that contains valuable information regarding pelvic pain and its treatment: www. physioforwomen.com.

PERSISTENT GENITAL AROUSAL DISORDER

Persistent genital arousal disorder (PGAD) is defined as persistent feelings of genital arousal occurring without an obvious precipitant and persisting for extended periods, despite one or more orgasms.[3] This disorder has only recently been identified and studied in women. Usually, women feel sexual arousal sensations as pleasurable and desired when in the context of sexual activity with a partner. However, PGAD may be triggered not only by sexual activity, but also by seemingly nonsexual stimuli or even no apparent stimulus at all. The signs of arousal are experienced as intrusive and unwanted, and the affected women report feelings of emotional and physical distress. The symptoms of PGAD include feelings of genital fullness and sensitivity which do not subside on their own or with orgasm.

Prevalence of PGAD is unknown. The majority of women who complain of this disorder are in relatively good health, well educated, and in long-term relationships. The causes of PGAD are still largely a mystery. Some theorize that PGAD may be linked to the use of or discontinuation of SSRI medication, such as Zoloft, Prozac, Lexapro, and others. Other theories have investigated possible central nervous system changes, such as post-injury or brain anomalies. Additionally, some theories are looking at vascular changes (pelvic congestion), peripheral neurological changes (pelvic nerve sensitivity or entrapment), and mechanical pressure against genital structures. Psychological changes have also been examined as a link to the etiology of PGAD. This disorder will continue to be studied, providing new information and treatment. A woman diagnosed with PGAD faces a difficult situation because the cause is unknown and may be a combination of the above-mentioned conditions.

Treatment can involve changing medications, identifying triggers that exacerbate the condition, pelvic massage, biofeedback, anesthetizing agents to numb the area, and psychological techniques of relaxation and support. There is a support group online at www.psas-support.com.

SENSATE FOCUS

We have mentioned the helpfulness of using sensate focus with the above sexual disorders. Sensate focus is sensual massage or comforting touch that is not meant to necessarily include orgasm or intercourse. Appendix C contains helpful information about sensate focus; we encourage you and your partner to read it and talk about trying some of the exercises.

C

SENSATE FOCUS

Masters and Johnson developed sensate focus exercises in the 1970s to help couples with performance anxiety. Sensate focus exercises are now often referred to as sensual exercises, non-demand pleasuring exercises, or caressing exercises and may be prescribed by a therapist or a health-care provider. The term "sensate focus" is used to highlight that the focus of the exercises is on physical and sensual sensations of touch and not simply on the goal of orgasm or intercourse. The purpose of sensate focus is the experience itself and it is not meant to be a form of foreplay leading necessarily to sexual intercourse. Sensate focus was designed to help reduce anxiety and to help couples learn about their sexual responses.

A couple engaging in sensate focus exercises might choose to refrain from intercourse so that all pressure and expectation is alleviated. By removing the "objective" of the encounter from intercourse alone, the couple can learn to heighten the awareness of a wide range of stimuli that can include all of the senses. Perhaps orgasm and intercourse are appropriate goals for some couples who are "prescribed" sensate focus exercises or who decide to try them on their own. This is fine, keeping in mind that performance- or goal-oriented sexual encounters can lead to a great deal of stress for some couples or individuals. It's helpful to talk this issue out thoroughly so that you know when or if it's advisable to attempt orgasm or intercourse.

The advantages of sensate focus are many. It can slow down the interaction so that the couple can feel present during the sexual encounter.
Sensate focus allows each person to concentrate on physical sensations
without feeling the expectation to proceed to intercourse or to achieve
orgasm. It removes the pressure to perform and can teach the participants about the body's responses to certain types of touch that may have
been avoided in the past.

In order to complete a sensate focus exercise, the couple needs about
thirty minutes of uninterrupted time. Each person takes a turn receiving
and giving touch without trying to produce a sexual response. When first
trying a sensate focus exercise, usually the genitals and breasts are not
touched or caressed. It's advisable to offer limited verbal feedback during
the session and to try to stay focused on physical and emotional sensations. Talking about the exercise afterward can help the couple explore
what was sensual and what might have been distracting. As the sensate
focus exercises advance (giving thirty minutes, on different occasions,
to each sensate focus activity), the couple can include the genitals and
breasts and possibly more verbal feedback during the session. The "hand-
guiding" technique can be incorporated, in which the receiver puts his or
her hand on top of the giver's hand to guide touch, indicating the type of
touch, the pressure, and other sensations the receiver finds enjoyable.

It's critical that the couple discuss these exercises fully so that neither
feels that the experience is "forced," but is instead enriching. If the couple has decided to refrain from orgasm or intercourse, but finds this is
anxiety provoking, it's important to discuss this with one another or with
a therapist. The point of sensate focus is to enhance self-understanding
regarding desire and arousal.

Depending upon the level of comfort with different forms of touch,
a couple can begin by simply holding hands and giving a hand massage. Partners could also begin with clothes on, kissing and touching in
nonsexual areas. Sensate focus can be a launch into the investigation of
touch and varying sensations. Often couples are accustomed to leading
directly into intercourse with minimal touching. Especially if sexual
discomfort, performance anxiety, or physical pain have developed, it's
a good idea to step back from the notion of intercourse and explore affectionate intimate touch again.

Imagine the comfort and relief you might feel to establish sensate focus exercises if you and/or your partner have found that sex has become

dysfunctional. You might be having pain with intercourse, experiencing discomfort with endometriosis, interstitial cystitis, or vaginismus. Or perhaps early ejaculation has caused so much anxiety that you're having erectile failure. Consider the feeling of relaxation that can be possible if you choose sensate focus, instead of struggling with a sexual difficulty, dreading sex, or avoiding sex altogether.

Sensate focus may be prescribed in certain steps, such as described in chapter 3; some issues need to be broken down into stages or gradual desensitization steps. You and your partner can also make this list of steps for whatever problem you may be having. To make this desensitization list, write down in your journal all the things that would lead up to the most anxiety-provoking activity or the activity that would present the dysfunctional concern (i.e., rapid ejaculation, delayed ejaculation, painful intercourse). Then set this list up in gradual increments, from least troubling to most troubling, and talk with your partner about trying each step with you. You will probably need to use the progressive muscle relaxation, also described in chapter 3, as you attempt these steps.

Here's an example of a desensitization list for someone struggling with vaginismus:

Least anxiety provoking to most:

- We're sitting, clothed, and kissing.
- We're lying together with our underwear on and talking about our love for one another.
- We're lying together in the nude, talking about what we love about one another.
- He's lying beside me and I'm touching him everywhere, except his penis.
- He's not erect, and he's touching my breasts, lying beside me.
- He's on top of me or I'm on top of him and he's caressing my breasts.
- He's watching me touch my clitoris and vulva.
- He's touching me with his fingers or mouth on my clitoris and vulva. And he has an erection.
- He's got an erection and is touching me around my vulva with his erect penis.
- He's got a hard erection and is about to enter me.

You can see from this list that the female with vaginismus will need to move very slowly from being completely in control to allowing increased intimate touching. Try this with your partner regarding any issues that are of concern for either of you. Then move very slowly with gentle and appropriate caressing so that there is increasing trust and comfort around whatever the sexual issue might be.

Sensate focus can be really sexy for a couple when the usual technique has become predictable, familiar, and mechanical. When dealing with sexual boredom and routine, find thirty minutes and try the following, wherever you and your partner feel comfortable:

- Give or receive a hand or foot massage. Use lotions and take your time.
- Lie on the bed with clothes on and kiss, cuddle, and rub one another, but stay away from goal-centered arousal techniques. Simply be present.
- Relax in the tub with your partner spooned in front of you and gently caress his or her torso and genitals.
- Explore one another's body while still wearing something sexy. Prolong going to intercourse; perhaps skip it altogether.
- Kiss your partner as you want to be kissed.
- Show your partner how you like to touch yourself to arousal.

We want to recommend some excellent websites and resources for learning more about massage and sensate focus.

www.dodsonandross.com
  Viva la Vulva: Women's Sex Organs Revealed
  Celebrating Orgasm: Women's Private Selfloving Sessions

www.HSAB.org
  A Heterosexual Couples Guide to Sexual Pleasure
  A Lesbian Couples Guide to Sexual Pleasure
  A Gay Male Couples Guide to Sexual Pleasure

www.sinclairinstitute.com
  Joy of Erotic Massage

www.alexanderinstitute.com

Ⓓ

HAVING THE "TALK"
WITH YOUR CHILDREN

Throughout this book, we have discussed how to talk about sex with many different people in our lives. What about talking to our kids about sex? If the sexual information we received was faulty, how do we ensure that our kids don't get the same messages that we got when we were children?

There are several areas to focus on when we talk to kids about sex:

- What is age-appropriate information for my child?
- What words will we use to discuss genitals?
- When is the best time to start talking to my child about sex?
- What values do I want to teach my child about sex?

When it comes to talking to kids about sex, the best time to start is from the very beginning. We are sexual beings at every age, and kids have sexual feelings. When kids are little, we teach them messages from the time they are born. Kids naturally ask questions and some-times the questions have to do with genitals, bodily functions, where babies come from, or other sexual matters. How do we talk about these things?

YOUNG CHILDREN

Use correct terminology to describe body parts. After all, we would never refer to an arm as anything but an arm. We don't want to give the child the impression that genitals are shameful. Furthermore, there may be times when adults need to understand what body part your child is referring to when they talk about their "yoohoo." A child might need to tell a teacher, doctor, or nurse that their genitals are hurt or sore. When we work with children in our practices, we see many kids who have suffered from different types of abuse. It is difficult to figure out what part of the body the child is referring to when they say "peach" or "winky."

So your toddler wants to know where babies come from. What is the correct response? Stay away from the stork, the hospital, or any other untruth or half-truth. It's really okay to say that a baby comes from "a special place moms have called a uterus." If you desire to include a more spiritual response, you might say, "God gave a special place to moms . . ." Give the answer, and then elaborate only if more questions follow. For instance, what if the child asks, "How did the baby come out?" An appropriate answer for a small child might be that "the mom's uterus pushes the baby out through the mom's vagina, which is shaped like a tunnel."

Kids ask all kinds of questions about their own bodies. A preschool-age boy might ask about why his penis gets hard. Simply reassure him that this is natural, that it happens to all boys, and that it will get soft again. This lets him know that his body is doing something normal and it's nothing he should be worried or ashamed about, as it happens to every boy.

Then there's the dilemma of masturbation. All children will eventually find their genitals, and when they do, they discover that rubbing the area feels really good. What do we say to our kids? The best thing to do is tell them that you know rubbing their penis or vulva feels good, but these are their private parts, so it should be done in private. Be sure not to move their hands away or tell them to stop. Explain to your children that if someone else touches their genitals, they should tell a parent or another adult.

AS CHILDREN GET OLDER

As children get older, the questions will get more challenging. Think about what you'll say before your child asks so that it's not a surprise and you'll be prepared with an answer. As with younger children, you'll want to answer the question in terms the child understands. Answer the question, only elaborating if your child wants more information.

Eventually, we all have to address the issue of intercourse. The best way to handle this is something like the following: "A mom's and dad's private places fit together just right. Something called sperm comes from the dad's penis and goes in the mom's vagina."

PRE-TEENS AND TEENS

Use teachable current events or television shows to open up the table for discussion. For example, a pregnancy in the family, such as that of an aunt or cousin, might be an occasion to ask your child what their understanding is of pregnancy. A show on television might address teen pregnancy or sexually transmitted infections (STIs). Use this opportunity to discuss how sex affects one's life and the importance of being responsible. Discuss birth control and safe sex, emphasizing that self-restraint is the only guarantee of avoiding STIs or pregnancy. Keep in mind that teenagers are going to experiment and explore their sexuality, and we need to discuss alternative, but safe, sexual expression.

HOW ABOUT VALUES?

Think about what your values are and what you want to teach your children about sex and relationships. The important thing is to talk about and relay your value message to your children, whether you tell them to wait until marriage, to wait for love, or to wait until after they graduate. Be sure to discuss that their bodies are their own, and when they (male or female) decide to have sex, it should be with someone who is respectful and cares about them and their well-being. Let them know that sex is a pleasurable experience and that having it with someone they trust can make it even more special.

More topics for "the talk":

- Anatomy—show your child an appropriate book or website that shows correct anatomy. Go over all the parts and the function of each part.
- Menstruation—talk to girls about this early so that they aren't shocked when they start menstruating.
- Nocturnal emissions (wet dreams)—boys need to know what is happening before it happens, so they don't think something is wrong. Hearing about this experience from other boys instead of his parents will give him the message that it's a secret and shameful.
- Erections—discuss the normalcy of erections and ways to handle spontaneous erections.
- Orgasms—explain what an orgasm is and how the body reacts.
- Sexual orientation—help your child understand what homosexuality and transsexuality are.

We know these are uncomfortable topics to discuss with your children. Keep in mind that whether or not you discuss them with your children, they will masturbate, have wet dreams, experience orgasms, and be confronted in some way with homosexuality or transgender issues. A parent is the best person to inform a child about sex. We can open a door that allows a child to come to us with important life questions in the future.

There are excellent websites in chapter 2 that can help describe these topics and others. Go to these websites with your children to help answer their questions.

NOTES

CHAPTER I

1. Helen Fisher, *Why We Love* (New York: Henry Holt and Company, 2004).

CHAPTER 2

1. Salvador Minuchen, *Family Kaleidoscope* (Cambridge, MA: Harvard University Press, 1984).

CHAPTER 3

1. David Finkelhor, "The International Epidemiology of Child Sexual Abuse," *Child Abuse and Neglect* 18 (1994): 409–17.
2. Wendy Maltz, *The Sexual Healing Journey: A Guide for Survivors of Sexual Abuse* (New York: Quill, 2001), 30.
3. Mike Lew, *Victims No Longer: The Classic Guide for Men Recovering from Sexual Child Abuse*, 2nd ed. (New York: Quill, 2004), 31.
4. Peter T. Dimock, "Adult Males Sexually Abused as Children: Characteristics and Implications for Treatment," *Journal of Interpersonal Violence* 3, no. 2 (June 1988): 203–21.

5. Paul Joannides, *Guide to Getting It On* (N.p.: Goofy Press, 2009).

6. Eliana Gil, *Outgrowing the Pain: A Book for and about Adults Abused as Children* (New York: Dell, 1983).

7. Ellen Bass and Laura Davis, *The Courage to Heal*, 3rd ed. (New York: HarperCollins, 1994).

8. Maltz, *The Sexual Healing Journey*.

9. Judith Herman, *Trauma and Recovery* (New York: Basic Books, 1997).

10. American Psychiatric Association, *Diagnostic and Statistical Manual of Medical Disorders*, 4th ed., text revision (Washington, DC: American Psychiatric Association, 2000).

11. Stephanie Buehler, "Childhood Sexual Abuse: Effects on Female Sexual Function and Its Treatment," *Current Sexual Health Reports* 5 (2008): 154–58.

12. American Psychological Association, *Answers to Your Questions: For a Better Understanding of Sexual Orientation and Homosexuality* (Washington, DC: American Psychological Association, 2008), www.apa.org/topics/soreintation.pdf.html (August 15, 2009).

13. Joe Kort, *Gay Affirmative Therapy for the Straight Clinician* (New York: W. W. Norton, 2008).

14. Ibid., 48.

CHAPTER 4

1. William H. Masters and Virginia Johnson, *Human Sexual Response* (Boston: Little, Brown, 1966).

2. Edward O. Laumann, John H. Gagnon, Robert T. Michael, and Stuart Michaels, *The Social Organization of Sexuality: Sexual Practices in the United States* (Chicago: University of Chicago Press, 1994).

3. Helen S. Kaplan, *The New Sex Therapy* (New York: Brunner/Mazel, 1974).

4. Rosemary Basson, "The Female Sexual Response: A Different Model," *Journal of Sex and Marital Therapy* 26, no. 1 (January–March 2000): 51–65.

5. Jennifer Berman and Laura Berman, *For Women Only: A Revolutionary Guide to Reclaiming Your Sex Life* (New York: Henry Holt and Company, 2001).

6. Michael E. Metz and Barry W. McCarthy, "The 'Good-Enough Sex' Model for Couple Sexual Satisfaction," *Sexual and Relationship Therapy* 22, no. 3 (August 2007): 351–62.

7. Lonnie Barbach, *For Each Other* (New York: Anchor Books, 2001).

CHAPTER 5

1. Sallie Foley, Sally A. Kope, and Dennis P. Sugrue, *Sex Matters for Women: A Complete Guide to Taking Care of Your Sexual Self* (New York: Guilford Press, 2002).

2. American Heart Association, *Sex and Heart Disease* (Dallas: American Heart Association, 2009), www.americanheart.org/presenter. jhtml?identifier=9239 (August 15, 2009).

3. Anne Katz, *Breaking the Silence on Cancer and Sexuality* (Pittsburgh, PA: Oncology Nursing Society, 2007).

4. Kairol Rosenthal, *Everything Changes: The Insider's Guide to Cancer in Your 20s and 30s* (Hoboken, NJ: Wiley and Sons, 2009).

5. Ibid., 54.

6. Katz, *Breaking the Silence.*

7. World Health Organization, *International Classification of Functioning Disability and Health* (Geneva: World Health Organization, 2001), www.who. int/icf (August 15, 2009).

8. Paul Joannides, *Guide to Getting It On*, 6th ed. (N.p.: Goofy Press, 2009).

9. Marita P. McCabe and George Talepores, "Sexual Esteem, Sexual Satisfaction, and Sexual Behavior among People with Physical Disabilities," *Archives of Sexual Behavior* 32, no. 4 (August 2003): 359–69.

10. Miriam Kaufman, Cory Silverberg, and Fran Odette, *The Ultimate Guide to Sex and Disability: For All of Us Who Live with Disabilities, Chronic Pain, and Illness* (San Francisco, CA: Cleis Press, 2007).

11. Stacy Tessler Lindau, L. Philip Schumm, Edward O. Laumann, Wendy Levinson, Colm A. O'Muircheartaigh, and Linda J. Waite, "A Study of Sexuality and Health among Older Adults in the United States," *New England Journal of Medicine* 357 (August 2007): 762–74.

12. Bernie Zilbergeld, *Better Than Ever* (Norwalk, CT: Crown House Publishing Company, 2004).

13. Peggy J. Kleinplatz, A. Dana Menard, Marie-Peirre Paquet, Nicolas Paradis, Meghan Campbell, Dino Zuccarino, and Lisa Mehak, "The Components of Optimal Sexuality: A Portrait of 'Great Sex,'" *Canadian Journal of Human Sexuality* 18, nos. 1–2 (2009): 1–13.

14. Helen Fisher, *Why We Love* (New York: Henry Holt and Company, 2004).

CHAPTER 7

1. Edward O. Laumann, John H. Gagnon, Robert T. Michael, and Stuart Michaels, *The Social Organization of Sexuality: Sexual Practices in the United States* (Chicago: University of Chicago Press, 1994).

2. Jennifer Berman and Laura Berman, *For Women Only: A Revolutionary Guide to Reclaiming Your Sex Life* (New York: Henry Holt and Company, 2001).

3. Michael E. Metz and Barry W. McCarthy, "The 'Good-Enough Sex' Model for Couple Sexual Satisfaction," *Sexual and Relationship Therapy* 22, no. 3 (August 2007): 351–62.

4. Laumann et al., *Social Organization*.

5. Wendy Maltz and Susie Boss, *Private Thoughts* (Novato, CA: New World Library, 2001).

6. Ibid.

7. Leanne Nicholls, "Putting the New View Classification Scheme to an Empirical Test," *Feminism and Psychology* 18, no. 4 (November 2008): 515–26.

8. Barry W. McCarthy and Emily McCarthy, *Rekindling Desire: A Step-by-Step Program to Help Low-Sex and No-Sex Marriages* (New York: Brunner-Routledge, 2003).

CHAPTER 8

1. John M. Gottman and Julie Schwartz Gottman, *Ten Lessons to Transform Your Marriage* (New York: Random House, 2006), 34.

2. Michael Bader, *Male Sexuality: Why Women Don't Understand It, and Men Don't Either* (Lanham, MD: Rowman & Littlefield, 2009), 60.

3. Wendy Maltz and Larry Maltz, *The Porn Trap: The Essential Guide to Overcoming Problems Caused by Pornography* (New York: HarperCollins Publishers, 2008), 43.

CHAPTER 9

1. Michael J. Bader, *Arousal: The Secret Logic of Sexual Fantasies* (New York: St. Martin's Press, 2002), 33.

2. Anne Semans, *The Many Joys of Sex Toys* (New York: Broadway Books, 2004).

3. Bernie Zilbergeld, *Better Than Ever* (Norwalk, CT: Crown House Publishing Company, 2004).

4. Janice Korff and James H. Geer, "The Relationship between Sexual Arousal Experience and Genital Response," *Psychophysiology* 20 (March 1983): 121–27.

5. Jennifer Berman and Laura Berman, *For Women Only: A Revolutionary Guide to Reclaiming Your Sex Life* (New York: Henry Holt and Company, 2001).

6. Michael E. Metz and Barry W. McCarthy, "The 'Good-Enough Sex' Model for Couple Sexual Satisfaction," *Sexual and Relationship Therapy* 22, no. 3 (August 2007): 351–62.

7. Talli Rosenbaum, "Pelvic Floor Exercises and Sex," www.physioforwomen.com (August 15, 2009).

8. Judy Kuriansky, *The Idiot's Guide to Tantric Sex* (New York: Alpha Books, 2004), 4.

CHAPTER 10

1. Barnaby Barratt and Marsha Rand, "'Sexual Health Assessment' for Mental Health and Medical Practitioners: Teaching Notes," *American Journal of Sexuality Education* 4 (2009): 16–27.

2. Jack Annon, *The Behavioral Treatment of Sexual Problems* (Honolulu, HI: Enabling Systems, 1974).

CHAPTER 11

1. Yvonne Fulbright, "Schools Shy Away from Sexuality Training," *New Physician* 56, no. 7 (October 2007): 1.

2. JoAnne Mick, Mary Hughes, and Marlene Cohen, "Sexuality and Cancer: How Oncology Nurses Can Address It BETTER," *Oncology Nursing Forum* 30, no. 2 (2003): 152–53.

APPENDIX A

1. Michael E. Metz and Barry W. McCarthy, *Coping with Premature Ejaculation: Overcome PE, Please Your Partner, and Have Great Sex* (Oakland, CA: New Harbinger, 2003).

2. Ibid.

3. Ibid.

4. Raymond C. Rosen, Rena Wing, Stephen Schneider, and Noel Gendrano, III, "Epidemiology of Erectile Dysfunction: The Role of Medical Comorbidity and Lifestyle Factors," *Urologic Clinics of North America* 32 (2005): 403–17.

5. Raymond C. Rosen, "Erectile Dysfunction: Integration of Medical and Psychological Approaches," in *Principles and Practice in Sex Therapy*, 4th ed., ed. Sandra Leiblum (New York: Guilford Press, 2007), 277–310.

6. Raymond C. Rosen, William A. Fisher, Ian Eardley, Craig Niederberer, Andrea Nadel, and Michael Sand, "The Multinational Men's Attitudes of Life Events and Sexuality (MALES) Study: Prevalence of Erectile Dysfunction and Related Health Concerns in the General Population," *Current Medical Research and Opinion* 20 (2004): 607–17.

7. Michael E. Metz and Barry W. McCarthy, *Coping with Erectile Dysfunction: How to Regain Confidence and Enjoy Great Sex* (Oakland, CA: New Harbinger, 2004).

8. Michael E. Metz and Barry W. McCarthy, "The 'Good-Enough Sex' Model for Couple Sexual Satisfaction," *Sexual and Relationship Therapy* 22, no. 3 (August 2007): 351–62.

9. Edward O. Laumann, John H. Gagnon, Robert T. Michael, and Stuart Michaels, *The Social Organization of Sexuality: Sexual Practices in the United States* (Chicago: University of Chicago Press, 1994).

10. Michael A. Perelman and David L. Rowland, "Retarded Ejaculation," *World Journal of Urology* 24, no. 6 (December 2006): 645–52.

APPENDIX B

1. Rosemary Basson, "The Female Sexual Response: A Different Model," *Journal of Sex and Marital Therapy* 26, no. 1 (January–March 2000): 51–65.

2. Nathan Seppa, "Viagra and Women," *Science News* 174, no. 4 (August 18, 2008): 1–2.

3. Sandra Leiblum, Candace Brown, and Jim Wan, "Persistent Sexual Arousal Syndrome: A Descriptive Study," *Journal of Sexual Medicine* 2 (2005): 331–37.

RESOURCES

BOOKS AND WEBSITES

General Sexuality

Bader, Michael. *Arousal: The Secret Logic of Sexual Fantasies.* New York: St. Martin's Press, 2002.

Britton, Patti. *The Art of Sex Coaching: Expanding Your Practice.* New York: W. W. Norton and Company, 2005.

Brown, Mildred L., and Stephen Braveman. *CPR for Your Sex Life: How to Breathe Life into a Dead or Dull Sex Life.* N.p.: BookSurge, 2007.

Buehler, Stephanie. *Sex and Passion: The Essential Guide.* Buehler Institute, 2009. www.thebuehlerinstitute.com/sexandpassion.htm (August 9, 2009).

Fisher, Helen. *Why We Love.* New York: Henry Holt and Company, 2004.

Fulbright, Yvonne. *Touch Me There! A Hands-On Guide to Your Orgasmic Hot Spots.* Alameda, CA: Hunter House, 2007.

Joannides, Paul. *Guide to Getting It On.* 6th ed. N.p.: Goofy Foot Press, 2009.

Komisaruk, Barry K., Carlos Beyer-Flores, and Beverly Whipple. *The Science of Orgasm.* Baltimore, MD: Johns Hopkins University Press, 2006.

McCarthy, Barry, and Emily McCarthy. *Discovering Your Couple Sexual Style.* New York: Routledge, 2009.

———. *Rekindling Desire: A Step-by-Step Program to Help Low-Sex and No-Sex Marriages.* New York: Brunner-Routledge, 2003.

Nelson, Tammy. *Getting the Sex You Want*. Beverly, MA: Quiver, 2008.

Perel, Esther. *Mating in Captivity*. New York: HarperCollins Publishers, 2006.

Semans, Anne. *The Many Joys of Sex Toys*. New York: Broadway Books, 2004.

Zoldbrod, Aline P., and Lauren Dockett. *Sex Talk: Uncensored Exercises for Exploring What Really Turns You On*. Oakland, CA: New Harbinger, 2002.

www.goodcleanlove.com—Certified Coop American Green Company that sells natural and organic green products for health and sexual enhancement.

www.HSAB.org—Health and Science Advisory Board: an interdisciplinary team of over forty leading academics, educators, theologians, and medical professionals worldwide, providing articles, DVDs, and virtual lectures.

www.nsrc.sfsu.edu—National Sexuality Resource Center, providing advice and information on sexuality (aging, faith, disability, education, gender, LGBTQI, etc.).

www.sexualhealth.com—A group of credentialed experts providing sexuality education (STIs, disabilities and chronic conditions, love and relationships, male and female sexuality, etc.).

Male Sexuality

Bader, Michael. *Male Sexuality: Why Women Don't Understand It and Men Don't Either*. Lanham, MD: Rowman & Littlefield, 2009.

Castleman, Michael. *Great Sex: A Man's Guide to the Secret Principles of Total-Body Sex*. New York: Rodale Press, 2004.

Hunter, Mic. *Abused Boys: The Neglected Victims of Sexual Abuse*. New York: Fawcett Books, 1990.

Lew, Mike. *Victims No Longer: The Classic Guide for Men Recovering from Sexual Childhood Abuse*. New York: HarperCollins, 2004.

Metz, Michael, and Barry McCarthy. *Coping with Erectile Dysfunction: How to Regain Confidence and Enjoy Great Sex*. Oakland, CA: New Harbinger, 2004.

———. *Coping with Premature Ejaculation: Overcome PE, Please Your Partner, and Have Great Sex*. Oakland, CA: New Harbinger, 2003.

———. *Men's Sexual Health: Fitness for Satisfying Sex*. New York: Routledge, 2008.

Milsten, Richard, and Julian Slowinski. *The Sexual Male: Problems and Solutions*. New York: W. W. Norton, 1999.

Moran, Martin. *The Tricky Part: A Boy's Story of Sexual Trespass, a Man's Journey to Forgiveness*. New York: Anchor Books, 2006.

Zilbergeld, Bernie. *The New Male Sexuality*. New York: Bantam Books, 1999.

www.malesurvivor.org—A website for male survivors of sexual abuse.

www.renewintimacy.org—Ralph and Barbara Alterowitz website providing articles and book recommendations for individuals with prostate cancer.

www.straightguise.com—A website for straight men who have sex with men and who question their sexual orientation and are not gay.

Female Sexuality

Barbach, Lonnie. *For Each Other: Sharing Sexual Intimacy*. New York: Anchor Books, 2001.

Berman, Laura. *Real Sex for Real Women*. New York: DK Adult, 2008.

Cass, Vivienne. *The Elusive Orgasm*. New York: Avalon Publishing, 2007.

Chalker, Rebecca. *The Clitoral Truth: The Secret World at Your Fingertips*. New York: Seven Stories Press, 2003.

Diamond, Lisa M. *Sexual Fluidity: Understanding Women's Love and Desire*. Cambridge, MA: Harvard University Press, 2008.

Foley, Sallie, Sally A. Kope, and Dennis Sugrue. *Sex Matters for Women: A Complete Guide to Taking Care of Your Sexual Self*. New York: Guilford Press, 2002.

Goodwin, Aurelie Jones, and Marc E. Agronin. *A Woman's Guide to Overcoming Sexual Fear and Pain*. Oakland, CA: New Harbinger, 1997.

Hall, Kathryn. *Reclaiming Your Sexual Self: How You Can Bring Desire Back into Your Life*. Hoboken, NJ: Wiley & Sons, 2004.

Heiman, Julia, and Joseph LoPiccolo. *Becoming Orgasmic*. New York: Simon & Schuster, 1992.

Karras, Nick. *Petals*. San Diego, CA: Crystal River Publishing, 2003.

Maltz, Wendy. *The Sexual Healing Journey: A Guide for Survivors of Sexual Abuse*. New York: HarperCollins, 2001.

Maltz, Wendy, and Susie Boss. *Private Thoughts*. Novato, CA: New World Library, 2001.

Ogden, Gina. *The Return of Desire: A Guide to Rediscovering Your Sexual Passion*. Boston: Trumpeter Books, 2008.

Paget, Lou. *How to Be a Great Lover: Girlfriend-to-Girlfriend Totally Explicit Techniques That Will Blow His Mind*. New York: Broadway Books, 1999.

Pertot, Sandra. *Perfectly Normal: Living and Loving with Low Libido*. New York: Rodale, 2005.

Sheehy, Gail. *Sex and the Seasoned Woman*. New York: Ballantine Books, 2006.

Sundahl, Deborah. *Female Ejaculation and the G-Spot*. Alameda, CA: Hunter House, 2003.

Waxman, Jamye. *Getting Off: A Woman's Guide to Masturbation*. Emeryville, CA: Seal Press, 2007.

www.balegoonline.org—Website providing the Pelvic Floor Educator (found under "Incontinence Urology Training"), which can help train the pelvic floor muscles and ensure that Kegels are performed correctly.

www.fsd-alert.org—The "new view" approach to female sexual problems.
www.ichelp.org—Interstitial Cystitis Association website.
www.pelvicpain.org—International Pelvic Pain Society's website.
www.physioforwomen.com—Talli Rosenbaum, urogynecological physiotherapist, provides information and articles regarding pelvic disorders at this website.
www.psas-support.com—Online support group for women with persistent genital/sexual arousal syndrome.
www.sexualityresources.com—Website for A Woman's Touch sexuality resource center, which contains sexual education, health information, and tasteful shopping for women and those who love them.
www.The-Clitoris.com—Visuals and articles about female anatomy.
www.twshf.org—The Women's Sexual Health Foundation website.
www.vaginismus.com—Website that explains diagnosis, symptoms, treatment of vaginismus.

Menopause

Caine-Francis, Dona. *Managing Menopause Beautifully: Physically, Emotionally, and Sexually*. Westport, CT: Praeger, 2008.
Northrup, Christiane. *The Wisdom of Menopause: Creating Physical, Emotional, and Mental Health during the Change*. New York: Bantam Books, 2006.
www.menopause.org—North American Menopause Society website.

GLBT Resources

Boylan, Jennifer Finney. *She's Not There: A Life in Two Genders*. New York: Broadway Books, 2004.
Chernin, Jeffrey. *Get Closer: A Gay Man's Guide to Intimacy and Relationships*. New York: Alyson Books, 2006.
Devor, Holly. *FTM: Female-to-Male Transsexuals in Society*. Bloomington: Indiana University Press, 1999.
Girshick, Lori, and Jamison Green. *Transgender Voices: Beyond Women and Men*. Lebanon, NH: University Press of New England, 2009.
Helminiak, Daniel A. *Sex and the Sacred: Gay Identity and Spiritual Growth*. Binghamton, NY: Haworth Press, 2006.
Hutchins, Loraine, and Lani Kaahumanu. *Bi Any Other Name: Bisexual People Speak Out*. New York: Alyson Books, 1994.
Jenson, Karol. *Lesbian Epiphanies: Women Coming Out in Later Life*. New York: Routledge, 1999.

Klein, Fritz. *The Bisexual Option*. 2nd ed. Binghamton, NY: Haworth Press, 1993.

Kort, Joe. *Gay Affirmative Therapy for the Straight Clinician: The Essential Guide*. New York: W. W. Norton, 2008.

———. *Ten Smart Things Gay Men Can Do to Find Real Love*. New York: Alyson Books, 2006.

———. *Ten Smart Things Gay Men Can Do to Improve Their Lives*. New York: Alyson Books, 2003.

Newman, Felice. *The Whole Lesbian Sex Book: A Passionate Guide for All of Us*. San Francisco, CA: Cleis Press, 2004.

Rose, Donna. *Wrapped in Blue: A Journal of Discovery*. Round Rock, TX: Living Legacy Press, 2003.

www.fishcantfly.com—Tom Murray, director and producer, explores the lives of gay men and women of faith as they recall their journeys to put their sexuality and spirituality in harmony.

www.heartscrackedopen.com—Tantra DVD for women who love women.

Sexuality and Aging

Block, Joel. *Sex over Fifty*. New York: Perigee Trade, 2008.

Fisher, Deirdre, and Diana Holtzberg. *Still Doing It: The Ultimate Lives of Women over Sixty*. New York: Avery, 2008.

Kliger, Leah, and Deborah Nedelman. *Still Sexy After All These Years? The 9 Unspoken Truths About Women's Desire Beyond 50*. New York: Perigee Trade, 2006.

Price, Joan. *Better Than I Ever Expected: Straight Talk about Sex after Sixty*. Emeryville, CA: Seal Press, 2006.

Sheehy, Gail. *Sex and the Seasoned Woman: Pursuing the Passionate Life*. New York: Ballantine Books, 2007.

Zilbergeld, Bernie. *Better Than Ever*. Norwalk, CT: Crown House Publishing Company, 2004.

Sexuality and Cancer

Katz, Anne. *Breaking the Silence on Cancer and Sexuality: A Handbook for Healthcare Providers*. Pittsburgh, PA: Oncology Nursing Society, 2007.

———. *Woman Cancer Sex*. Pittsburgh, PA: Oncology Nursing Society, 2009.

Laken, Virginia, and Keith Laken. *Making Love Again: Hope for Couples Facing Loss of Sexual Intimacy*. Sandwich, MA: Ant Hill Press, 2002.

Mulhall, John. *Saving Your Sex Life: A Guide for Men with Prostate Cancer*. Munster, IN: Hilton Publishing, 2008.

Perlman, Gerald, and Jack Drescher. *A Gay Man's Guide to Prostate Cancer*. New York: Haworth Medical Press, 2005.

Rosenthal, Kairol. *Everything Changes: The Insider's Guide to Cancer in Your 20s and 30s*. Hoboken, NJ: Wiley & Sons, 2009.

Silver, Marc. *Breast Cancer Husband: How to Help Your Wife (and Yourself) through Diagnosis, Treatment, and Beyond*. New York: Rodale, 2004.

Relationship Matters

Chapman, Gary. *The Five Love Languages: How to Express Heartfelt Commitment to Your Mate*. Chicago: Northfield Publishing, 2004.

Glass, Shirley. *Not "Just Friends": Rebuilding Trust and Recovering Your Sanity after Infidelity*. New York: Free Press, 2003.

Gottman, John, and Nan Silver. *The Seven Principles for Making Marriage Work*. New York: Three Rivers, 1999.

Lusterman, Don-David. *Infidelity: A Survival Guide*. Oakland, CA: New Harbinger, 1998.

McCarthy, Barry, and Emily McCarthy. *Getting It Right the First Time: Creating a Healthy Marriage*. New York: Brunner-Routledge, 2004.

Sexuality and Porn

Maltz, Wendy, and Larry Maltz. *The Porn Trap*. New York: HarperCollins, 2008.

Schneider, Jennifer, and Burt Schneider. *Sex, Lies, and Forgiveness: Couples Speaking on Healing from Sex Addiction*, 3rd ed. Tucson, AZ: Recovery Resources Press, 2004.

Weiss, Robert. *Cruise Control: Understanding Sexual Addiction in Gay Men*. Los Angeles: Alyson Books, 2005.

Weiss, Robert, and Jennifer Schneider. *Untangling the Web: Sex, Porn, and Fantasy Obsession in the Internet Age*. New York: Alyson Books, 2006.

Sex and Disability

Baer, Robert. *Is Fred Dead? A Manual on Sexuality for Men with Spinal Cord Injuries*. Pittsburgh, PA: Dorrance Publishing, 2004.

Blackburn, Maddie. *Sexuality and Disability*. Woburn, MA: Butterworth-Heinemann, 2002.

Kaufman, Miriam, Cory Silverberg, and Fran Odette. *The Ultimate Guide to Sex and Disability: For All of Us Who Live with Disabilities, Chronic Pain, and Illness*. San Francisco, CA: Cleis Press, 2007.

Kroll, Ken, and Erika Klein. *Enabling Romance: A Guide to Love, Sex, and Relationships for the Disabled*. Baltimore, MD: No Limits Communication, 2001.
www.comeasyouare.com—Website with disability resources and sex toy information.

Spirituality and Sex

Anand, Margo. *The Art of Sexual Ecstasy: The Path of Sacred Sexuality for Western Lovers*. Los Angeles: Jeremy Tarcher, 1989.
Carrellos, Barbara. *Urban Tantra: Sacred Sex of the Twenty-First Century*. Berkeley, CA: Celestial Arts, 2007.
Kuriansky, Judy. *The Idiot's Guide to Tantric Sex*. New York: Alpha Books, 2004.
Ogden, Gina. *The Heart and Soul of Sex: Making the ISIS Connection*. Boston: Trumpeter Books, 2006.
Savage, Linda E. *Reclaiming Goddess Sexuality: The Power of the Feminine Way*. Carlsbad, CA: Hay House, 1999.

DVDs

The following DVDs include information regarding sexual technique. The authors are not endorsing these websites; please use your own judgment when accessing any of these sites.

www.alexanderinstitute.com—Website with DVDs regarding sexual techniques.

www.dodsonandross.com—Betty Dodson and Carlin Ross—website with DVDs for self-pleasuring.

www.fishcantfly.com—Tom Murray, director and producer, explores the lives of gay men and women of faith as they recall their journeys to put their sexuality and spirituality in harmony.

www.healthysex.com—Wendy Maltz's website with DVDs for relearning touch after sexual abuse.

www.heartscrackedopen.com—Tantra DVD for women who love women.

www.HSAB.org—Health and Science Advisory Board website; contains DVDs about sensate focus for heterosexual, lesbian, and gay couples.

www.sexsmartfilms.com—This site promotes positive sexual education and literacy. Sexsmartfilms preserves, archives, and showcases films addressing sexual health issues. The films are both contemporary and classic.

www.sinclairinstitute.com—Website with instructive and informative DVDs.

ADULT TOY SITES

www.bettersex.com
www.comeasyouare.com—Disability resources and sex toy information.
www.goodvibrations.com
www.mypleasure.com
www.pureromance.com—General shopping section plus a product line for
cancer patients.
www.sinclairinstitute.com

EROTICA

Blue, Violet. *Best Women's Erotica*. San Francisco, CA: Cleis Press, 2008.
Friday, Nancy. *Forbidden Flowers: More Women's Sexual Fantasies*. New
York: Pocket Books, 1993.
Maltz, Wendy, ed. *Intimate Kisses: The Poetry of Sexual Pleasure*. Novato, CA:
New World Library, 2001.
———. *Passionate Hearts: The Poetry of Sexual Love*. Novato, CA: New World
Library, 2007.
Tyler, Alison. *Afternoon Delight: Erotica for Couples*. San Francisco, CA: Cleis
Press, 2009.
———. *Frenzy: 60 Stories of Sudden Sex*. San Francisco, CA: Cleis Press, 2008.
www.cleansheets.com
www.erotica-readers.com/ERA/index.htm
www.scarletletters.com

BIBLIOGRAPHY

Amen, Daniel. *Sex on the Brain*. New York: Harmony Books, 2007.

American Heart Association. "Sex and Heart Disease." *American Heart Association*, 2009. www.americanheart.org/presenter.jhtml?identifier=9239 (August 15, 2009).

American Psychiatric Association. *Diagnostic and Statistical Manual of Medical Disorders*, 4th ed., text revision. Washington, DC: American Psychiatric Association, 2000.

American Psychological Association. "Answers to Your Questions: For a Better Understanding of Sexual Orientation and Homosexuality." *American Psychological Association*, 2008. www.apa.org/topics/soreintation.pdf.html (August 15, 2009).

Annon, Jack. *The Behavioral Treatment of Sexual Problems*. Honolulu, HI: Enabling Systems, 1974.

Bader, Michael. *Arousal: The Secret Logic of Sexual Fantasies*. New York: St. Martin's Press, 2002.

———. *Male Sexuality: Why Women Don't Understand It and Men Don't Either*. Lanham, MD: Rowman & Littlefield, 2009.

Barbach, Lonnie. *For Each Other: Sharing Sexual Intimacy*. New York: Anchor Books, 2001.

Barrett, Barnaby, and Marsha Rand. "'Sexual Health Assessment' for Mental Health and Medical Practitioners: Teaching Notes." *American Journal of Sexuality Education* 4 (2009): 16–27.

Bass, Ellen, and Laura Davis. *The Courage to Heal*, 3rd ed. New York: Harper-Collins, 1994.

Basson, Rosemary. "The Female Sexual Response: A Different Model." *Journal of Sex and Marital Therapy* 26, no. 1 (January–March 2000): 51–65.

Berman, Jennifer, and Laura Berman. *For Women Only: A Revolutionary Guide to Reclaiming Your Sex Life*. New York: Henry Holt and Company, 2001.

Berman, Laura. "The Sex Ed Handbook: A Comprehensive Guide for Parents." Oprah.com, 2009. media.oprah.com/lberman/talking-to-kids-about-sex-handbook.pdf (July 31, 2009).

Buehler, Stephanie. "Childhood Sexual Abuse: Effects on Female Sexual Function and Its Treatment." *Current Sexual Health Reports* 5 (2008): 154–58.

Dimock, Peter T. "Adult Males Sexually Abused as Children: Characteristics and Implications for Treatment." *Journal of Interpersonal Violence* 3, no. 2 (June 1988): 203–21.

Finkelhor, David. "The International Epidemiology of Child Sexual Abuse." *Child Abuse and Neglect* 18 (1994): 409–17.

Fisher, Helen. *Why Him? Why Her?* New York: Henry Holt and Company, 2009.

———. *Why We Love*. New York: Henry Holt and Company, 2004.

Foley, Sallie, Sally A. Kope, and Dennis Sugrue. *Sex Matters for Women: A Complete Guide to Taking Care of Your Sexual Self*. New York: Guilford Press, 2002.

Fulbright, Yvonne. "Schools Shy Away from Sexuality Training." *New Physician* 56, no. 7 (October 2007): 1.

Gil, Eliana. *Outgrowing the Pain: A Book for and about Adults Abused as Children*. New York: Dell, 1983.

Glass, Shirley. *Not "Just Friends": Rebuilding Trust and Recovering Your Sanity after Infidelity*. New York: Free Press, 2003.

Gottman, John, and Nan Silver. *The Seven Principles for Making Marriage Work*. New York: Three Rivers, 1999.

Hastings, Ann. *Treating Sexual Shame: A New Map for Overcoming Dysfunction, Abuse, and Addiction*. Northvale, NJ: Jason Aronson, 1998.

Herman, Judith. *Trauma and Recovery*. New York: Basic Books, 1997.

Joannides, Paul. *Guide to Getting It On*. 6th ed. N.p.: Goofy Foot Press, 2009.

Kaplan, Helen S. *The New Sex Therapy*. New York: Brunner/Mazel, 1974.

Katz, Anne. *Breaking the Silence on Cancer and Sexuality: A Handbook for Healthcare Providers*. Pittsburgh, PA: Oncology Nursing Society, 2007.

———. *Woman Cancer Sex*. Pittsburgh, PA: Oncology Nursing Society, 2009.

Kaufman, Miriam, Cory Silverberg, and Fran Odette. *The Ultimate Guide to Sex and Disability: For All of Us Who Live with Disabilities, Chronic Pain, and Illness*. San Francisco, CA: Cleis Press, 2007.

Kleinplatz, Peggy J., A. Dana Menard, Marie-Peirre Paquet, Nicolas Paradis, Meghan Campbell, Dino Zuccarino, and Lisa Mehak. "The Components of Optimal Sexuality: A Portrait of 'Great Sex.'" *Canadian Journal of Human Sexuality* 18, nos. 1–2 (2009): 1–13.

Korff, Janice, and James H. Geer. "The Relationship between Sexual Arousal Experience and Genital Response." *Psychophysiology* 20 (March 1983): 121–27.

Kort, Joe. *Gay Affirmative Therapy for the Straight Clinician: The Essential Guide*. New York: W. W. Norton & Company, 2008.

Kuriansky, Judy. *The Idiot's Guide to Tantric Sex*. New York: Alpha Books, 2004.

Laumann, Edward O., John H. Gagnon, Robert T. Michael, and Stuart Michaels. *The Social Organization of Sexuality: Sexual Practices in the United States*. Chicago: University of Chicago Press, 1994.

Leiblum, Sandra, ed. *Principles and Practice in Sex Therapy*. 4th ed. New York: Guilford Press, 2007.

Leiblum, Sandra, Candace Brown, and Jim Wan. "Persistent Sexual Arousal Syndrome: A Descriptive Study." *Journal of Sexual Medicine* 2 (2005): 331–37.

Lew, Mike. *Victims No Longer: The Classic Guide for Men Recovering from Sexual Childhood Abuse*. New York: HarperCollins, 2004.

Lindau, Stacy Tessler, L. Philip Schumm, Edward O. Laumann, Wendy Levinson, Colm A. O'Muircheartaigh, and Linda J. Waite. "A Study of Sexuality and Health among Older Adults in the United States." *New England Journal of Medicine* 357 (August 2007): 762–74.

Maltz, Wendy. *The Sexual Healing Journey: A Guide for Survivors of Sexual Abuse*. New York: HarperCollins, 2001.

Maltz, Wendy, and Susie Boss. *Private Thoughts*. Novato, CA: New World Library, 2001.

Maltz, Wendy, and Larry Maltz. *The Porn Trap*. New York: HarperCollins, 2008.

Masters, William H., and Virginia Johnson. *Human Sexual Response*. Boston: Little, Brown, 1966.

McCabe, Marita P., and George Talepores. "Sexual Esteem, Sexual Satisfaction, and Sexual Behavior among People with Physical Disabilities." *Archives of Sexual Behavior* 32, no. 4 (August 2003): 359–69.

McCarthy, Barry, and Emily McCarthy. *Rekindling Desire: A Step-by-Step Program to Help Low-Sex and No-Sex Marriages*. New York: Brunner-Routledge, 2003.

Metz, Michael, and Barry McCarthy. *Coping with Erectile Dysfunction: How to Regain Confidence and Enjoy Great Sex*. Oakland, CA: New Harbinger, 2004.

———. *Coping with Premature Ejaculation: Overcome PE, Please Your Partner, and Have Great Sex.* Oakland, CA: New Harbinger, 2003.

———. "The 'Good-Enough Sex' Model for Couple Sexual Satisfaction." *Sexual and Relationship Therapy* 22, no. 3 (August 2007): 351–62.

Mick, JoAnne, Mary Hughes, and Marlene Cohen. "Sexuality and Cancer: How Oncology Nurses Can Address It BETTER." *Oncology Nursing Forum* 30, no. 2 (2003): 152–53.

Minuchen, Salvador. *Family Kaleidoscope.* Cambridge, MA: Harvard University Press, 1984.

Nicholls, Leanne. "Putting the New View Classification Scheme to an Empirical Test." *Feminism and Psychology* 18, no. 4 (November 2008): 515–26.

Perel, Esther. *Mating in Captivity: Unlocking Erotic Intelligence.* New York: Harper, 2006.

Perelman, Michael A., and David L. Rowland. "Retarded Ejaculation." *World Journal of Urology* 24, no. 6 (December 2006): 645–52.

Rosen, Raymond C. "Erectile Dysfunction: Integration of Medical and Psychological Approaches." In *Principles and Practice in Sex Therapy*, 4th ed., ed. Sandra Leiblum, 277–310. New York: Guilford Press, 2007.

Rosen, Raymond C., William A. Fisher, Ian Eardley, Craig Niederberer, Andrea Nadel, and Michael Sand. "The Multinational Men's Attitudes of Life Events and Sexuality (MALES) Study: Prevalence of Erectile Dysfunction and Related Health Concerns in the General Population." *Current Medical Research and Opinion* 20 (2004): 607–17.

Rosen, Raymond C., Rena Wing, Stephen Schneider, and Noel Gendrano, III. "Epidemiology of Erectile Dysfunction: The Role of Medical Comorbidity and Lifestyle Factors." *Urologic Clinics of North America* 32 (2005): 403–417.

Rosenbaum, Talli. "Pelvic Floor Exercises and Sex." www.physioforwomen. com (August 15, 2009).

Rosenthal, Kairol. *Everything Changes: The Insider's Guide to Cancer in Your 20s and 30s.* Hoboken, NJ: Wiley & Sons, 2009.

Semans, Anne. *The Many Joys of Sex Toys.* New York: Broadway Books, 2004.

Seppa, Nathan. "Viagra and Women." *Science News* 174, no. 4 (August 18, 2008): 1–2.

World Health Organization. "International Classification of Functioning Disability and Health." *Geneva: World Health Organization*, 2001. http://www.who.int/icf (August 15, 2009).

Zilbergeld, Bernie. *Better Than Ever.* Norwalk, CT: Crown House Publishing Company, 2004.

INDEX

ABOUT THE AUTHORS

Libby Bennett is a clinical psychologist in practice for more than twenty years. She holds a doctorate in clinical psychology from Forest Institute in Springfield, Missouri. Dr. Bennett is a certified sex therapist through AASECT and is a past member of its board of directors. She is an adjunct instructor of human sexuality at Forest Institute. Dr. Bennett is a frequent speaker to community and professional groups.

Ginger Holczer is a clinical psychologist in practice for more than ten years. Dr. Holczer graduated from Forest Institute in Springfield, Missouri, with a doctorate in clinical psychology. She is a member of AASECT and presents to business and community groups. She has been an adjunct supervisor of graduate students at Forest Institute.